REVISED & EXPANDED

HAND
Reflexology
KEY TO
PERFECT HEALTH

MILDRED CARTER
& TAMMY WEBER

PRENTICE HALL PRESS

Library of Congress Cataloging-in-Publication Data

Carter, Mildred.
   Hand reflexology : key to perfect health / Mildred Carter and
Tammy Weber. — Rev. ed.
      p.   cm.
   ISBN 0-7352-0128-5 (pbk.). — ISBN 0-13-016230-2 (preprint)
   1. Reflexology (Therapy)   2. Hand.   I. Weber, Tammy.   II. Title.
RM723.R43C373   2000
615.8′22—dc21   99-38511
                                                            CIP

This book is a reference manual based on research by the authors. All techniques and suggestions are to be used at the reader's sole discretion. The opinions expressed herein are not necessarily those of, or endorsed by, the publisher. Information is to be used as a guide to help restore balance within the body, so it can heal itself. The directions stated in this book do not constitute the practice of medicine. Nor are they intended as claims for curing a serious disease and are in no way to be considered as a substitute for consultation with a duly licensed doctor.

Printed in the United States of America

Photographs by: Keith Jensen; Jennifer Rodgers; Tammy Weber
Illustrations: Zina Saunders

10 9 8 7 6 5 4 3 2 1

ISBN 0-7352-0128-5 (p)

PRENTICE HALL PRESS
Paramus, NJ 07652

On the World Wide Web at http://www.phdirect.com

Also by Mildred Carter

Healing Yourself with Foot Reflexology
Body Reflexology: Healing at Your Fingertips

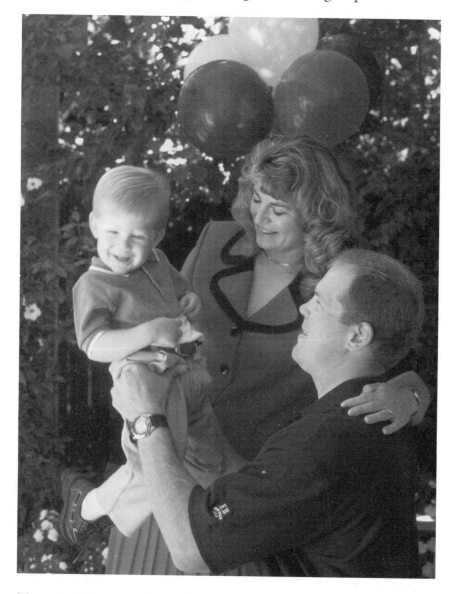

Photo 1: Kick up your heels. You are about to discover what reflexology can do to improve your life!

Acknowledgments

Special appreciation goes to Dr. Lloyd B. Rapp, N.D., Sutherline, Oregon; Dr. H. A. Hagan, D.C., Cottage Grove, Oregon; and Dr. J. P. Schaller, D.C., Paradise, California, for their counsel and help. Also thanks to Dr. R. C. Wilborn, D.C., of Health Research, Mokelumne Hill, California, for giving permission to use material from several of his books. Thanks to Dr. James Brandt for his part in making it possible for me to continue my research into this ancient healing art of Reflexology. Thank you, doctors, for your cooperation and help in compiling this book.

Tammy and I would like to thank all those pictured in the book, including Clayton Barnes, Steve Brigance, Cindy Carney, Natalie Davey, Wayne L. Davey, Wesley M. Davey, Marisa C. Galvez, Cindy J. Gray, Christa L. Green, Lauren M. Green, Shirlee D. Hayden, Frank E. Hurling, Virginia H., Brian Weber, Kevin Weber, Sandra J. Weber, Sherryl Weber, Gordon Weber, Quintin Weber, and Dawna M. Williams. May your reflections of enthusiasm and willingness to share, touch the world with enlightenment.

We are grateful to Stirling Enterprises for their cooperation in supplying materials for some of the photos.

In addition, we thank all of you who use the powerful healing forces of Reflexology to help yourselves and others. Honor the gift of each new day, and enjoy your future in perfect health.

Foreword

It gives me much pleasure to add a few lines to Mildred Carter's fascinating book on reflexology. My attention to this field and its therapeutic value was drawn by my learned friend Aslam Effendi, who, among other things, is a student of the Carter school and has been giving convincing demonstrations of the techniques outlined in this book for laymen. For example, abnormal conditions in the body show up in the hands and feet; and no such reflexes are found in healthy people.

Many centuries back, the Chinese physicians discovered acupuncture, and something similar was practiced in the Indo-Pakistan subcontinent. But it was only in the beginning of this century that some medical pioneers in the West improved on the techniques of the ancient oriental physicians by developing Reflexology (or western-type acupressure). And today, Reflexology can certainly prove an effective weapon in the hands of physiotherapists and the medical profession generally. Perhaps it was the pioneering work of Reflexologists that inspired Elizabeth Kenny to develop her technique to combat poliomyelitis, and thus gain world recognition despite bitter opposition from the medical profession.

As a physician and scientist, I have learned one very important lesson—and that is to be always a humble and curious student. Therefore, Mildred Carter and pioneers like her who are trying in their own humble way to unveil some of the vast mysteries of the healing art, deserve our respectful attention.

Z. Hussain, M.B., B.S.
Consulting Physician
Pakistan

Preface

This book is written in response to many requests from people who were introduced to the wonderful healing powers of reflexology as described in my earlier book, *Healing Yourself with Foot Reflexology*. Some found it difficult to use the self-help techniques on their feet for various reasons. Therefore, many have requested detailed information on pressure points in the hands.

Hands contain the same reflexes as the feet, but locating the "miracle buttons" that bring prompt relief from many ailments requires its own rules. Simple but effective manipulation of the hands has brought renewed health and vitality to many.

For those who have not read my previous book, it was necessary to repeat some of the information given there so this book, limited to hand reflexology, would be as complete as possible in itself.

Hand reflexology is so simple that it can be used anywhere by anyone—including athletes, students, sportspeople, caregivers, desk workers, physical workers, homemakers, children, and travelers. By following a few simple rules, reflexology can be used indoors or out, and in any occupation or activity, with perfect safety.

The reader is cautioned, however, that there are some conditions that may require the attention of a medical doctor or chiropractor. When this is the case, common sense dictates that such care should be sought.

Mildred C.

Brief History of Reflexology

Although the principles of reflexology have been known for centuries, with the advance of medical science, this practice was slowly discarded for newer innovations. The new methods were not always better, and required considerable experimentation not only with animals, but also with humans.

In 1913, Dr. William Fitzgerald rediscovered reflexology. He brought it to the attention of the medical world. In an article in *The Health Counselor,* published in Southern California, he states, "Zone therapy [as it was called] has been practiced and taught by some of the most noted doctors in America."

Dr. Joe Selby Riley (M.D., M.S., D.C., N.D.), of Washington, D.C., was a well-known exponent of reflexology. He charted many of the reflex points, and said, "The scope of the science of Zone Reflex (Reflexology) is almost unlimited. Great physicians who have investigated it fully made the claim that it is the greatest ally yet found to their work. Side by side with other great therapies, zone therapy will stand in the march of science and progress."

Reflexology has been retained in health centers by professional reflexologists. However, the general public is so exposed to pills, salves, ointments, tranquilizers, and surgery on offending organs, that the average person looks askance at the principle of working a reflex in the hands, or feet, to treat an ailing organ far distant in the body.

Reflexology is one of the most miraculous examples of using nature's own healing methods for maintaining the body and keeping it in peak condition. It requires no pills, drugs, tranquilizers, or mutilating surgery; can be self-administered with perfect safety, anywhere or anytime; and is used to help people of all ages.

The vital life force of the body circulates along pathways, and we can tap it at an estimated 800 points on the body. It is not necessary to know all of these points because the hands, as well as the feet, contain "reflex buttons" that are connected to all organs and glands.

When these reflex centers are worked correctly, they send a stimulating surge of new vigor to the corresponding part of the body, often alleviating problem conditions instantly and with no aftereffects such as we frequently suffer from medications. We are correcting imbalance in this primary flow and thereby helping nature do the healing.

This book shows you this "push button" method of reflexology with photographs, illustrations, charts, and easy-to-follow reflex techniques.

I constantly search for new methods of natural healing, and when I find one that is better than the positive and simple methods of reflexology, I will bring that method to you.

You need no longer live in fear of so-called incurable diseases. I believe that *nothing is incurable*. Diseases are the result of malfunctioning cells and imperfection of body tissues due to unnatural elements of living. Just turn to Nature and give her a chance to put your body chemistry back into normal performance by rebuilding perfect cells and new healthy tissues for your whole body.

How This Book Came to Be Written

It seems that I was born with a desire to help the sick and injured. As long as I can remember, I was rescuing and doctoring animals and birds and even bugs.

When I was very young, I remember rescuing prairie dogs that my father had gassed or poisoned. They were a great nuisance on the ranches, and the farmers were trying to exterminate them. I was gathering all the sick ones and doctoring them back to health until my father found my "clinic."

When I was about seven, I experienced a cure of the general weakness I had suffered from since early babyhood. No one knew what it was. When we moved to California, I met some children eating garlic. I couldn't seem to get enough of it. My poor mother was an understanding person and let me eat all I wanted even though she couldn't stand me near her because of the strong garlic odor. I was never sick again after that "garlic binge." I have since studied the wonderful healing powers of garlic and herbs. I think this experience has always stayed with me and slanted my interest toward other natural systems of cures for various illnesses.

When my husband was stricken with a heart attack in his early 30's, no doctor knew what to do for him. They knew very little about heart disease at that time. So I turned to prayer, studied diet where I could, and he had a very quick recovery. That is when I wrote my first book, *The Power of Thought*. When my husband passed away eight years later from virus pneumonia, the doctors said that by all laws of nature he should never have lived through the heart attack he had suffered years earlier.

I thought of studying to be a medical doctor but decided against it. If I did that, I would know only what doctors know. So I devoted my life to studying all phases of natural healing, of which there are many. But, to date, I have not found any method of physical healing that equals the simple, natural, and safe way to heal that *reflexology* offers. This is a method of healing that anyone can use on themselves or their family in complete safety with the most remarkable results.

AMAZING QUICK RECOVERIES

In my years of practicing reflexology, since the 1950s, I have never gotten over being totally amazed at the quick relief people received from so many ailments. It was as if I pushed a magic button to instant health, in many cases.

People would come into the office doubled over with pain and feeling completely hopeless. Most were convinced that such a simple thing as working and pressing certain points in the hands and feet could not possibly help. Nevertheless, a spouse, parent, or neighbor had insisted that they come. Oh, how enlightened I was by the amazed look on their faces when the pain actually stopped, sometimes within seconds!

REFLEXOLOGY SEEMS LIKE A MIRACLE

It gave me great satisfaction to watch people recuperate under my very eyes in just a short time, some taking longer than others, of course. Mr. A. came to me for treatments for over five years, not because he had anything the matter with him after the first few sessions, but because he liked the feeling of vitality and well-being that he felt after each treatment. He brought his mother from a great distance on many occasions, just to make sure she remained in good health.

These reflexology treatments are in no way miraculous, although they may seem that way. They merely open the channels so that the normal healing process can be speeded up by supplying more energy to the right places, thus aiding Nature in her work of repairing your body.

A good, full flow of water cannot run through a clogged or rusty pipe. The pipe must be cleaned of all obstructions to get the full flow of water through. This is true of your veins, the nerves, and the network of invisible energy channels.

TESTIMONIALS PROVE REFLEXOLOGY
RESTORES HEALTH

I can give you not hundreds, but thousands, of case histories I receive through the mail from people all over the world telling me of the wonderful results they are getting by using the simple method of reflexology. The following unsolicited testimonials are typical samples.

Reflexology Saved Us from a Lot of Needless Pain

Dear Mildred,

I have been your student since 1985. I bought my first book then, when I was teaching nutrition and started teaching your methods to my students also. My husband, bless his heart, knows your latest book by heart.

I can't thank you enough, you have saved us many a doctor bill, and from a lot of needless pain. We are retired now, and I am teaching my senior friends your methods. They thank me every day. They say, "I didn't know I could help myself," or "I'm so glad to know more about my body." You are the one who deserves all our thanks, if it wasn't for you we would all be in the dark about how wonderful our bodies are.

Bless you.

Love, K. W., California

Reflexology Saved My Life

Dear Mrs. Carter,

You concluded your "Body Reflexology" book with: "I have not written this book for you to read and cast aside. I want it to be put to daily use for yourself, your loved ones and your neighbor." The art of healing is a God-given gift, and He could not have bestowed this rare gift to a more selfless person. Through your three books on Feet, Hand and Body Reflexology, you have indeed made one of the greatest contributions to those who have been plagued with ill health the world over.

I have read and re-read them, and now I am studying them, chapter by chapter, as a bedtime routine, for, in a nutshell, reflexology has saved my life. From 1980 until March 1984, I was like a man waiting for death. I suffered through a string of ailments, diabetes, stomach ulcer, severe gastric pains, stress, arthritis, and insomnia . . . until I was warded at the Specialist Centre, a private hospital. And, of course, my monthly medical bills kept mounting . . .

My prayers were answered when a Chinese broth-seller showed me a foot reflexology chart and a book written in the Chinese language. I couldn't read Chinese, so he showed me the points on my feet to press. As my stomach trouble was my main problem then, he showed me the nerve point for the stomach on my foot. He instructed me to press on it. I did, and phew! I felt an acute pain at the particular spot on my foot, and the man confirmed that I had stomach trouble, all right.

The man told me to massage this spot, to rub out the pain every night before I go to bed. I did just that. That was the beginning of the road to my improved health. That, too, was the beginning of my all-consuming interest in reflexology.

It never occurred to me then that there could be books, in English, on reflexology. So I followed the broth-seller's instructions. I spent 20 minutes every night massaging the reflex zone of the stomach and, wonder of wonders, I no longer felt the pain. Three months later when I went to the doctor for my usual blood test for diabetes, the doctor recorded a drop of the sugar level from 320 mg to 155 mg. The doctor reduced my Daonil tablets from three to one. How the massaging of the stomach reflex zone could improve my diabetes, I did not know, then, anyway.

It was only later that I found out that the reflex zones for the duodenum and the pancreas were located near the stomach reflex zone. I realized then that while massaging the stomach reflex zone, I must have rubbed the other two zones and benefited from the result. My stomach and my diabetes had improved beyond what was expected.

Then, I came across your Foot Reflexology book. And for the first time since I first heard of the word REFLEXOLOGY, I knew I had found the book I had been looking for. So I went searching for more of your books and discovered the other two. You are definitely an authority on the subject. Your books certainly widened my perspective on reflexology. Now my workout includes massaging my palms and other parts of my body.

Having gone through so much suffering caused by this ailment and that, I have also recommended to ailing friends, colleagues, relatives, and neighbors to read all your books and use the healing magic of reflexology.

With Best Regards, yours faithfully,

Mr. Bobby C., Malaysia

How Reflexology Saved My Marriage

Dear Mrs. Carter,

Recently I pulled your book *Helping Yourself with Foot Reflexology*, off the library shelf to read, as I thought it might be interesting. I cannot begin to tell you what foot reflexology has already done for my life. I have spent many dollars and much mental anguish trying to regulate my female cycles, with no relief. Not only with the help of your book did I succeed in that, I have also saved my marriage.

I was diagnosed with a thyroid condition five years ago. I hemorrhaged a year and a half ago, and they told me it had nothing to do with my thyroid. After reading your book, I see indeed they are connected, as are the other glands. Now I am diligently working on getting myself back in order. The order that I am restoring to my body has brought my hormone level back to where it should be. I finally have other emotions in my body besides resentment and stress. I can actually feel love and joy.

That is how my marriage was saved. We are now trying to conceive a second child with the help of reflexology. I am planning on learning as much as I can and taking my studies to a higher level. I would like to work with people and use my knowledge as a service to others. Thank you very much for putting your knowledge in a book and making it available for others.

Sincerely,

P. M., New York

I Want to Share This "Miracle" with Those Who Need It

Dear Ms. Carter,

I have read your book *Body Reflexology* and I am totally amazed by how reflexology has helped me and those I have shared it with. Reflexology could be so beneficial to everyone and I would love to become a certified reflexologist and share this "miracle" with those who need it. Thank you for passing on your knowledge of this great "Treasure," and enlightening those of us fortunate enough to have read your books.

Sincerely,

J. W., New York

Reflexology Proves Doctors Wrong

Dear Mildred,

I am one of your fans and a true believer in reflexology. When I started this, they were getting ready to do an exploratory on me. The doctors told me because I was the youngest of 14 children (my mother was 45, and a diabetic when I was born and her body had been stripped of nutrition) that I would never feel good. . . . Well . . . can you believe, with your help, I proved them wrong. I am now 76 years old and going strong.

I have had breast surgery on both breasts, complete mastectomies, and other problems all my life. I felt terrible until I found your book on hand reflexology. Since then, I have purchased your book on feet, and now, your wonderful new book on body reflexology. I thank God for you every day. I cannot begin to tell you how many others I have helped with reflexology.

Thanks,

Mrs. D.M., Virginia

Reflexology and Nutrition Helped Overcome M.S.

Dear Mildred and Tammy,

A thousand blessings to you both for the production of a stupendous book. It has been a source of reassurance, and a wealth of knowledge. I had multiple sclerosis 21 years ago and my dear aunt did reflexology on my then-paralyzed body. I felt sensations in my shoulder area so we continued, and along with Adell Davis's book on nutrition, I did overcome this grave disease. I had to make many changes and a huge desire to overcome this ugly affliction. Life was good for about 19 years and then I ended up with myasthenia gravis. So I am now on my way out of that one. Your book has been a Godsend and it is paying off. I am truly grateful! Thank you for your book, and your time.

Sincerely,

D. S., Michigan

Reflexology Helped Me Rebound to Recovery

I am a 63-year-old nurse of 40-plus years, have been on disability, though I still work some. I have had numerous surgeries for arthritis, hysterectomy, and cancer. Now water retention and obesity are my biggest problems. I do not think (I know) I would not be here now if God had not worked a miracle! I have always believed that God has a cure for every disease. Pray for my continued improvement. Keep up the good work.

Sincerely,

G. T., Kentucky

Many Are Inspired to Use Reflexology

Mildred, you are a pioneer in reflexology who so many others and I admire. I would like to write a note for your new book, so that readers will know what a sharing person you are. This is from my heart and very sincere:

Mildred Carter is the first author to put the word *reflexology* in a book. It was in the title *Helping Yourself with Foot Reflexology*. Her philosophy is that everyone has the right to help themselves, or to receive help from another, through *natural* healing. Caring that others may benefit from her research is her passion.

Mildred's books are easy to understand. The clear illustrations and photographs make learning fun. When I meet people, even if English is a second language, they have her books, or have read and learned from them.

Thirty years ago when I started in Reflexology, Mildred Carter's books were very important, and to this day, her books are upgrading our need for knowledge. I am the co-founder of the Foot Reflexology Awareness Association. We have the opportunity to work with all kinds of people at health shows, marathons, and police games. We talk with people from all occupations, such as chiropractors, massage therapists, beauty operators, and persons just using the books to help themselves and their families. It never ceases to amaze me, all of these people have Mildred's books, and because of her, they became inspired and continue to pursue reflexology.

I was inspired 20 years ago to start a reflexology class based on Mildred's published work. I have used many of the pressure points obtained from her books to help relieve stress from my clients. I am sure this new revised book on Hand Reflexology, will be something everyone will want to learn from, use, and have in their home library.

James E. Ingram, FRAA, Mission Hills, California

Excellent Health at Seventy-seven

Ms. Carter,

Read your book *Body Reflexology.* Powerful! Along with prayer, it is keeping this old priest in excellent health at 77. Having used your advice for years, I find there is no need to visit doctors.

Thanks,

Sr. T. O., Hawaii

You can see why I want to give everyone the natural healing methods of reflexology. By the simple technique of pressing reflex buttons on your hands, body, or feet, you can activate a vital life force in all parts of your body. You can also use reflexology on someone else if you wish, for renewed magnetic energy. This will replenish health and delight you and your loved ones with a fuller, happier, healthful life.

Mildred Carter

Table of Contents

What This Book Will Do for You

Centuries ago, man mapped out a healing energy that circulates through the body on specific pathways. This energy we call "life force" or "vital energy." This force can be "tapped" at more than 800 points. This book shows you how to tap this healing current to bring natural and prompt relief from practically all your aches and pains, chronic or acute, by the simple process of working the "reflex buttons" located in your hands. These buttons are connected to all your glands, organs, and body systems.

The diagrams and photographs in these pages fully illustrate the techniques of reflexology. Simple self-help steps show how the various reflexes "signal" the presence of a malfunction in some gland or organ in the body. Clear instructions are given on how to send a surge of healing energy for prompt relief of a condition, merely by pressing and working the reflex connected to it. This method of restoring the body to normal functioning involves no expense, no special equipment, no drugs or medication. The results are amazingly fast, bringing relief often in a matter of seconds.

A glance at the Table of Contents will indicate the wide range of situations for which reflexology has been used to obtain beneficial results. Reflexology not only cures specific ailments but can be used to keep you in good health and help build resistance to attacks of disease. In addition, the method often detects health problems before they become serious. You will learn how to reduce health-destroying mental and physical tensions and regain youthful energy.

1

Reflexology is a simple technique that can be applied any time and practically anywhere. For instance, if you are suffering from a headache while attending a meeting, you can quickly stop the pain without anyone being the wiser.

Alternatively, you can take a "reflex break" for a fast boost of energy, in your office, while at a sports event, and even when you are on vacation or visiting friends.

This book also contains case histories of people whom I have encountered in my years of practice in the healing art of reflexology, as well as testimony from medical doctors who have recognized these natural healing properties. In addition, there are letters received from all over the world telling of personal experiences and recovery from illnesses through reflexology.

Reflexology is nature's "push button" secret for dynamic living, abundant physical energy, vibrant health, better living without pain, retaining youthful vigor, and enjoying life to the fullest—as is our birthright. By keeping this book within easy reach for reference when confronted with a health problem, you too can get all these benefits and even more.

THE VALUE OF GOOD ENERGY FLOW

A basic philosophy was explained in ancient medical books that health is dependent upon the balance and maintenance of harmony within the body.

To obtain this balance there must be a free and unimpeded circulation of energy flowing through the body's organs.

The aim of reflexology is to break down the blockage and restore the free flow of energy or life force through these invisible channels.

In studying the relation between acupuncture, not only of the Chinese, but from its use in other countries as well, we learn that the traditional medicine is based on a belief that the blood circulation follows the flow of energy. This energy circulates freely in an endless cycle from the main organs through the channels beneath the skin. If it is blocked at some point, the circulation is impaired. This blockage results in a deficient oxygenation of the tissues around the affected area and throws the body off balance. This imbalance produces malfunctioning not only of the tissues surrounding it, but, if not corrected, spreads to related organs nearby.

Naturalogists show that civilized man's environment and habits make his blood either the sparkling river of life or the stagnant stream of death.

As the toxins of the cells accumulate in the blood, due to environment and faulty habits, the body becomes flooded, shocked, and poisoned by its own excrement.

HOW YOU CAN GET INSTANT RELIEF WITH REFLEXOLOGY

You can readily see how to get instant relief when certain points in your hands or feet receive reflex stimulation. The crystals or blockages within the energy channels are being loosened and flushed out, thus allowing the life force to resume its free and natural flow through the channels. This encourages the body to swing back into its normal balance, so harmony and health are again established.

It is so simple when one knows how it works. It is like running fresh water into a muddy, stagnant pool. As soon as there is a continuous supply of clean water, the pool becomes sparkling and clear, full of life and beauty.

It is just this simple for you to start your fresh supply of renewed life forces circulating in your body, for a renewal of sparkling health!

Reflexology and Acupuncture

Reflexology and acupuncture come from an ancient art of healing; they are related and based on the same principle of healing. Where the Chinese insert needles in certain points of the body to treat illness, we of the western world use our fingers to press similar vital stimulating points, with comparable results. We are activating the vital life force and sending instant healing forces to malfunctioning parts of the body, even though these obstructed parts are far removed from the points that are being manipulated.

Several dignitaries have viewed acupuncture during visits to China; they have been quite impressed. Doctors there told them, "We treat the body as a whole, while western medicine treats the symptoms. They do not get at the cause and it's a vicious, never ending circle."

Health is in your hands. As explained in my previous book on foot reflexology, there is no portion of your wonderfully constructed feet which does not have its part to play in reflexology. I will say the same for your even more important wonderfully constructed hands. They also give you a unique way to health with the use of reflexology.

Reflexology Is a Natural Method of Healing

"Zone Therapy is scientific, subjectively and objectively," says W. D. Chesney, M.D. "That is to say that a patient using zone therapy (reflexology) knows he is getting results, and others see that he has improved.

"There is no substitute, and never will be a substitute for the trained eye, near, nose, and the sense of touch—the fingers. It is mainly with the fingers that the healer palpates as well as exerts them in zone therapy (reflexology). In medical school I learned the salient facts about reflexology. That is, that stimulation in one part of the human body often produced symptoms at far distant areas."

By using our fingers to search out and press on certain reflex buttons in the hands and the feet, we are learning to apply a simple and harmless method of healing—a method that can stop pain in all parts of the body almost instantly, with no physical or psychological harm of any kind.

Reflexology Can Be Used by Anyone

Reflexology can be used safely by anyone, from small children to the very elderly. I know of several young children who are experts in giving a reflex treatment with very good results.

I have letters from people in their 70's, 80's, and 90's who are not only using reflex techniques on themselves with great benefit, but also on others. Can you imagine the joy of these senior citizens when they can actually help stop the pain of their ailing friends; to watch their faces as their suffering subsides after a few minutes of pressing tender reflex buttons on their hands.

Imagine the relief they feel knowing how to stop their own pains as soon as they feel them coming on, and knowing that in many cases they are putting an end to the cause of the pain forever, with no more need of drugs or medication. What a wonderful world this will be when everyone learns how to use the marvelous magic of healing reflexology!

Acupuncture versus Reflexology: The world is looking to Chinese acupuncture at the present time. It seems that many are turning to needles for help in their despair of suffering from all kinds of diseases and ailments which the conventional doctors can't seem to cure. Let us learn to use our safe western style of pressing reflexes with the fingers instead of with needles. Results are just as good when used according to the simple directions given in this book.

Dr. Frank Mayo says:

> We are gravely concerned over the premature application of acupuncture to Americans for the relief of pain during surgery. A potentially valuable technique that has been developed over thousands of years in China is being hastily applied with little thought to safeguards or hazards. If acupuncture is applied indiscriminately, severe trauma (shock) could result in certain patients.

While Chinese therapists have expressed caution against premature use of *acupuncture,* many of our medical experts have used and recommended the use of *reflexology.* They have even taught their patients to use it on themselves with the full knowledge that there was no danger or harmful effects from the use of these natural techniques.

THE TRUE PHYSICIAN

In *A Lecture Course to Physicians,* George Starr White, M.D., writes, "A *real physician* will not hesitate to use any method that will relieve the sick. A *real quack* is one who will hesitate to use or recommend any method to relieve the sick, unless it is sanctioned by some governing board."

Giving someone a license to "heal the sick" does not make that person a physician. Christ was a *true physician,* and Bible records show that He did heal the sick. Records do not show that His license was given by a power higher than God.

What He did have was divine love, which radiated a vital life force. It filled the body, mind, and spirit of those who came to Him for help with vibrant energy that activated a healing response in every cell.

Reflexology should not be subject to manmade restrictions. It is a natural method, which is free for all to use on themselves, or others, to relieve pain and suffering. Reflexology is the key to perfect health. Please take this key and use it generously.

What a Medical Doctor Had to Say about Reflexology

Edwin Bowers, M.D., a well-known medical critic and writer, after a long, thorough investigation wrote a popular article regarding Dr. Fitzgerald's work in order that the public might be made aware of the new method of ridding themselves of pain. He called it *Zone Therapy.* Today we call it *Reflexology.*

He wrote, "The fact that today Zone Therapy is probably known more widely throughout the United States and all places where magazines and newspapers are printed than any other single method of therapy, proves that the foundation of the work is solid."

He wrote later, "One of the most disgraceful blots on the pages of organized medicine, or what is popularly known as 'The Medical Trust,' is the fact that they have apparently, in every way possible, tried to hinder the spread of the gospel of Zone Therapy. Because it was likely to educate the people into methods of *self-treatment,* they became *alarmed* and in various ways they have heaped abuse upon those who practice this method." And so it is today.

WHY REFLEXOLOGY WORKS TO BRING HEALTH BENEFITS

We are so conditioned to the need for pills, surgery, and special treatments for ailments that many people are somewhat skeptical about the effectiveness of such a simple method as reflexology. There are, of course, any number of theories about how or why it does work.

For instance, we are told by Alice Bailey that the "esoteric" body is really a network of fine channels that are component parts of one interlacing fine cord, one portion of this cord being the magnetic link which unites the physical and "astral" bodies, and which is broken at the time of death. This etheric web, of which we are a part, is composed of the intricate weaving of this vitalized "cord."

Thus we can easily see why massaging the reflexes to help nature open channels of health to any and all parts of the body is so positive, and why it cannot fail if applied properly. Reflexology not only helps nature open up these channels when congested *but also sends a supply of "prana," the magnetic vital life force of the universe charging through these channels like healing shock waves.* No wonder we have instant relief in so many cases of pain!

I hope you can see the simplicity of using reflexology and why it has to give some benefit to everyone who uses it, as it stimulates the *Golden Cord of Life* within you.

All of nature's ways are simple to use once we understand them.

Do Not Be Confused about Your Health

The more you read, the more you hear, the more confused you become. Every book, every lecturer, and every authority on health gives you a different answer, often contradictory. They will all point out their different special roads to glorious health.

Optimum health and freedom from disease start with correct and reliable information: information that has been verified by many, by people like you, people who have affirmed its worth by putting it to use; information from doctors who have demonstrated its value enough to use it in their practice.

I am giving you information so that you can use this art of natural healing to help yourself prevent premature aging and live longer in good health and freedom from disease.

Reflexology is not confusing, nor is it contradictory in any form. In this simple, easy-to-use, harmless, yet scientific way to health, you can learn how to stop pain all over your body. And in many cases, relief comes in a matter of seconds.

Although your situation is precarious and at times seems hopeless, your self-preservation instinct tells you not to give up.

People who are turning back to nature are experiencing the joys of regained health with little or no expense involved. *Natural health is free.*

CHAPTER 2

Step-by-Step Guide to Hand Reflexology Charts

Let us briefly study the reflexology charts of the hands, to get acquainted with the position of reflexes and their corresponding relation to the vital parts of the body. All diagrams of organs graphically shown in the hand charts represent their *reflex areas.*

I have purposely drawn diagrams of the organs and glands in the body very small, in order to place them all in the limited space of the hand. This will make it easier for you to identify the specific reflex area. Remember that the body is three dimensional, not flat like the charts.

HAND REFLEXOLOGY IS CONVENIENT TO USE

Reflexology to the hands has proven to be very convenient, especially for those who cannot comfortably reach their feet. We can use hand reflexology anywhere. It is suitable to use when traveling, and most appropriate when visiting friends. Many choose to use hand reflexology rather than the foot reflex methods, as hands are available anytime of the day or night.

Quite frequently, both hand and foot reflexology is used together for beneficial health maintenance. Reflexology is gaining popularity not only with therapists, but also with professional and physical workers who take time during their coffee or lunch breaks to use reflex techniques to renew energy or calm nerves.

Many athletes enjoy the stimulation of reflexology before competition starts. Caregivers at nursing homes use reflexology every day to give their seniors the caring touch of reflexology that also helps restore circulation; parents and partners enhance their loved ones' general health weekly; and the list goes on and on. People everywhere are benefiting from the rewards of reflexology.

Of course, there may be acute conditions that require the services of a medical doctor, and certain diseases that require special medications. The reader is cautioned to seek such professional help when the need is apparent.

Nature has provided the body with an astounding capacity to heal itself. It is up to each of us to take an active role in learning what the body needs to function properly. Reflexology is not intended as a substitute for medical care. It is a natural process of encouraging the body's own systems to rebalance and repair. The following charts are easy to understand. You will be referring to them often as you study the forthcoming chapters, so learn them well.

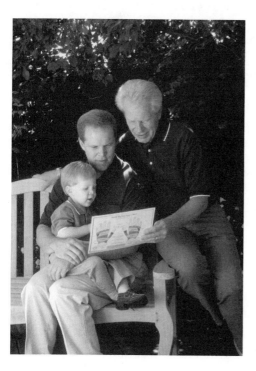

Photo 2: Reflexology charts will help you locate various reflex points when you need them.

VISUAL GUIDE TO THE ORGANS AND GLANDS

PINEAL GLAND
HYPOTHALAMUS
PITUITARY GLAND
BRAIN STEM

THROAT–THYROID–PARATHYROID–TONSILS

THYMUS

LUNGS

BRONCHIAL

HEART

SOLAR PLEXUS
DIAPHRAGM
ADRENALS

LIVER

GALL BLADDER

DUODENUM

SPLEEN
PANCREAS
STOMACH

TRANSVERSE COLON

ASCENDING COLON

ILEO-CECAL VALVE

APPENDIX

KIDNEYS

SMALL INTESTINE

DESCENDING COLON

SIGMOID COLON

BLADDER

RECTUM

Right Side   **Left Side**

Chart A: The amazing human body is wonderfully designed; it is a well-organized living entity that builds itself. It regulates its own functions, and remarkably repairs itself when hurt. Each organ and gland is designed to perform a particular task. There are reflex points in the hands that correspond to every part of the body. Learning about the body will be to your advantage when using hand reflexology.

HAND REFLEXOLOGY CHART (PALMS)

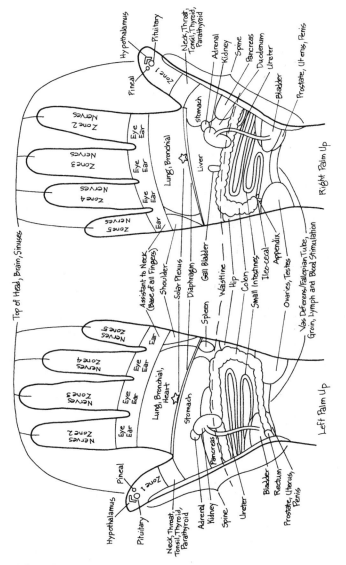

Chart B: This chart shows how to find reflex areas in your palms. Hold both hands out in front of your chest, with palms facing you. Keep in mind that reflexes in the right hand correspond to the right side of the body, and the left hand to the left side. The waistline on each hand represents the location of the waistline on the body. You will be referred to this chart often, as the palms are where we do most of our hand reflex work.

HAND REFLEXOLOGY CHART (BACK OF HANDS)

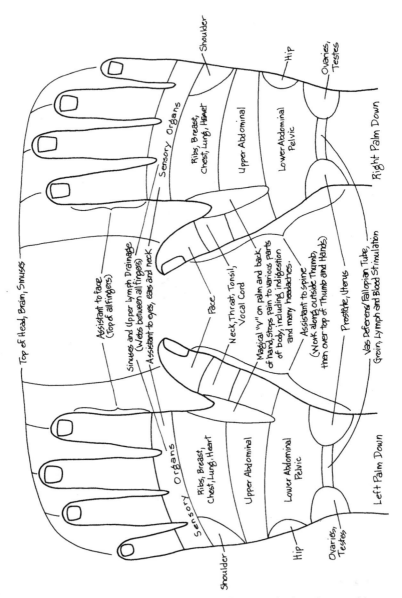

Chart C: By holding the hands in front of you with thumbs touching each other, you will be looking at what we call the back of our hands. By working these pressure points you will be fine-tuning basic reflex areas that are in the same zone, or same division as those in the palm.

HOW ENERGY CIRCUITS ARE ACTIVATED THROUGH THE HANDS

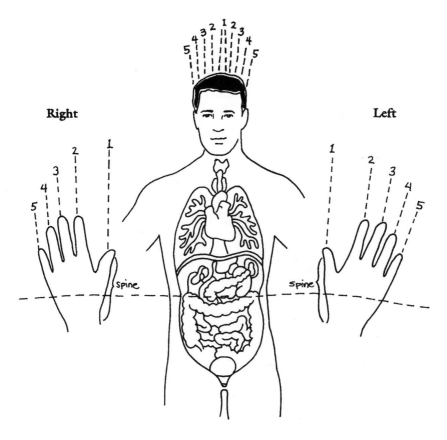

Chart D: Reflex stimulation will help clear pathways so the functional nerve energies have the power needed to reach all organs and glands. Good circulation helps ward off potentially harming health problems and creates the natural free flow of life surging through the body, for a natural balance and harmony. A complete reflex workout to all ten zones will encourage circulation to all systems for a renewal of sparkling health.

TEN ENERGY ZONES

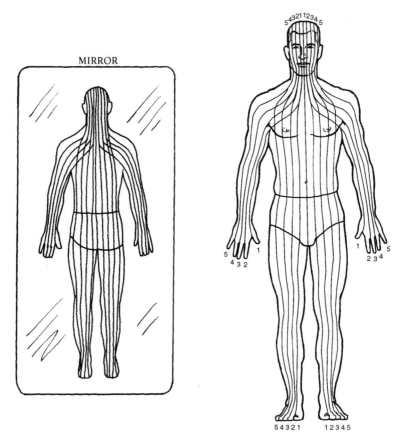

Chart E: This zone therapy chart shows the body divided into ten vertical zone pathways, five on each side of the body, one for each finger and each toe. All numbered zones extend the length of the body, from head to toe. In addition, every zone continues through the body, from the front to the back. These invisible zone lines are merely *clues* to help you locate specific reflexes to certain areas in the body.

EXPLANATION OF THE ENERGY ZONE CHART

When pressure is applied to a reflex area at the end of a zone, it stimulates a subtle force of nature's healing energy. As tiny nerve impulses clear away blockages, vital energy can flow freely through the whole body, encouraging a healthy balance.

Zone 1:   You will notice how line one goes down through the center of the head, then continues down the nose, mouth, neck and throat, and extends on down the spine. It includes the inside of the legs through the ankle reflexes and on down to the big toe. It also crosses over to and down the arm to the end of the thumb. Pain felt in any part of zone one can be helped by merely exerting pressure on thumbs or big toes.

Zone 2:   This zone is a little to the left, and to the right, of the spine. It also runs longitudinally through the head, neck, corner of the eye, corner of the nose, the teeth, and extends down the body to the second toe. Follow this zone down the arm, and notice it ends at the tip of the second finger.

Zone 3:   Note how this zone is a little more to the side of the head. It travels through the middle of each eye and follows on down through the body, ending with the third finger on each hand, and the third toe on each foot.

Zone 4:   This zone travels near the outer edge of the head and moves down the body to the leg and on down to the fourth toe, also moving down the arm and ending at the fourth fingertip.

Zone 5:   Follow zone five down the outer ear and the outer side of the face, down the outer side of the body, to the little toe. Notice how it travels down the shoulder and side of arm to the end of the little finger.

Analyzing the Zone Chart

You can see how the flow of this vital life energy is stimulated in different areas of the body when you use a rolling pressure on certain reflex points in the hands, fingers, feet, or toes.

For instance, pressure on the thumb will send an invigorating flow of circulation through the energy pathway of zone one.

Eye troubles can be helped by pressure exerted on the second, third, and fourth fingers.

As we follow on down, see how internal organs such as the stomach, kidneys, intestines, and colon are stimulated by pressure on certain reflexes in the palms of your hands.

You can also consider the simplicity of how a firm steady pressure on a specific reflex point controls pain within individual zones.

It may be easier for you to find the reflexes that correspond to the part of the body you are interested in helping by visually looking at Chart D on page 13. Now run imaginary zone lines down through the chart. Notice how each line follows through a definite part of the body.

Do not be discouraged if the charts seem a little complicated at first. Just keep referring to them, and before you know it, they will all be set in your mind. Remembering where the reflex areas are located is very important, because there will be many occasions when you will be away from home and not have your book with you just when you need it.

DIVISIONS OF THE BODY AND HANDS

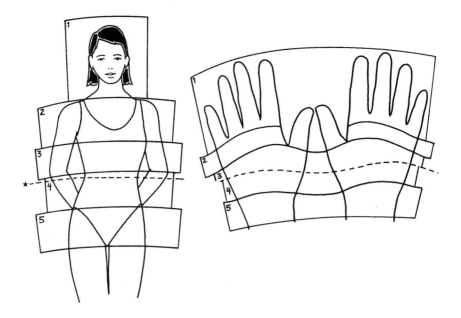

Chart F: Invisible divisions give us a better understanding of the body's regions, and how they correspond to the divisions on the hands.

1. Reflexes in the thumbs and fingers activate brain chemicals, and calm nerves. They also stimulate circulation to other parts of the head, such as the sinuses.

Reflexes at the base of thumbs and fingers channel to the sensory organs, such as nose, eyes, ears, and neck.

2. In the upper part of hands (on back side and palms) are reflexes that send healing energies to the chest and heart area.

3. Region three of the hands corresponds to areas in the upper abdomen.

★ The waistline, across both hands, matches up with the waistline of the body.

4. Reflexes in the heel of hands are counterparts to the lower torso of the body.

5. Reflex areas near the wrist coincide with the pelvic region.

GUIDE TO HAND REFLEXOLOGY CHARTS

Those of you who have my other two reflexology books, *Healing Yourself with Foot Reflexology* and *Body Reflexology, Healing at Your Fingertips,* will already be familiar with the body charts. It will be easy for you to familiarize yourself with the corresponding reflexes in the hands.

For instance, notice how the thumbs correspond to the head, as in the foot reflexology book, the big toes corresponded to the head. Note the position of the pituitary gland in the head in Chart A, page 10, and then look at the reflex to the pituitary gland in the center of the thumb in Chart B, page 11. The pituitary gland in the head will be stimulated by working the corresponding reflex in the thumb. Since this gland is located near the center of the head, you will work the reflex to it in both the left and the right thumb.

In review: Looking at Chart A, you see where the organs and glands are located in the body. To find a particular reflex, look at the other charts to see within which zone, division, or part of the hand that organ's or gland's corresponding reflex is.

Let us refer to the eye and ear reflexes on your hand charts. We see that they are just below the fingers, and since we have an eye and an ear on each side of the head, there will be reflexes on each hand. Fingers in the right hand will have reflexes to the right eye and ear, and fingers in the left hand will have the reflexes to the left eye and ear.

Recognize how the liver is located on the right side of the body, and the reflex to the liver is on the right hand. The spleen is on the left side of the body; on the charts, you see the reflex to the spleen in a corresponding area on the left hand.

The appendix is on the right side of the body, just below where the small intestine connects to the large intestine, under the liver. The corresponding reflex to the appendix is on the right hand, below the liver reflex.

You should now be getting an idea of how the positions of reflexes in the hands correlate to the locations of organs and glands in the body.

SUMMARY OF CHARTS

By studying these charts, you will get a fuller understanding of your body and the corresponding reflexes in your hands. Study them until you have the locations of the organs and glands somewhat established in your mind, in accordance with the reflex to each one.

After studying the charts, you can understand how pressing and correctly working all the reflexes in your hands will stimulate the whole body. You will not be treating just one congested area. You will be sending a flow of the energetic universal forces that created you charging throughout your entire system. This healing energy will help encourage the body to deal with specific health situations, and in many cases, return it to optimal functioning.

Easy-to-Use Hand Reflexology Techniques

The technique of working reflexes is to use the thumb or the fingers to press into the flesh over the reflex button you are trying to stimulate. You will press the thumb or fingers into the flesh deeply enough to feel the bone or muscles underneath. *You do not rub the skin.*

You may use a press-and-rotate movement on one spot, or "walk" your thumb or fingers over the hand, searching out sore spots. You will be amazed at how many you will find. Work each point for a few seconds, and move on. Keep the tender spots in mind, and return to them later. It will be best for you to sit in a relaxed position in a comfortable chair while learning your hand reflexology skills.

Structure of a reflexology point: Reflex animation feels good against the skin. However, the real power of reflexology works *beneath* the skin. Working the reflex area *under* the skin with a pressing-rolling motion activates healing energy waves that travel through the body, invigorating and renewing connective tissue, and restoring supportive cells.

As invisible radio waves travel through the air, the stimulation of reflex points causes energy waves to travel through the body. These chemical energy waves help improve circulation and bring nutritive oxygen to cells, helping to mend and rejuvenate the body.

Holding firm pressure on a reflex area *beneath* the skin causes it to heat up. The warmth triggers the release of endorphins, the neurochemicals that ease pain, thus bringing comfort to the body. Once pain is relieved, nerves will relax and the body can function peacefully.

SIMPLE GUIDELINES FOR USING REFLEX PROCEDURES

It will be a lot easier for you to learn reflexology if you start out using familiar techniques. Here you will learn to use your thumbs and fingers correctly, one for pressure and the other for support.

This technique will contribute to the overall efficiency of your reflex work. When reflexology is done properly, it relaxes nerves, provides considerable relief from various discomforts, and reestablishes internal balance to accelerate recovery time from illness. Your reflex work will be fun and easy to do once you learn these simple procedures.

How to Work Reflexes with Your Thumbs

Using your thumb properly will contribute to the overall efficiency of your reflex work.

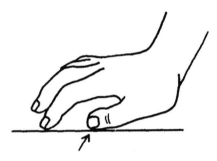

Illustration 1a: Place your hand down lightly on this book. Notice the *inside edge of your thumb* is touching the page. This is the "working" part of your thumb.

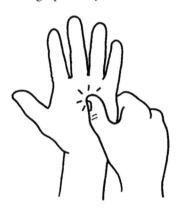

Illustration 1b: Slightly bend thumb at first joint, and use the "working edge" to reach deep reflex points. Thumbnails must be well trimmed.

How to use the press-and-rotate method: Use the working edge of your thumb to press-and-rotate on a reflex point. The fingers are used as leverage on the opposite side of the hand. Use a light, pressing, circular movement on the reflex for a moment, let up pressure, then press-and-rotate again, at a deeper level, for a few seconds. This approach works well on almost all reflex areas, and you can even use it when pinpointing a very small reflex point, such as the pituitary, spleen, or appendix.

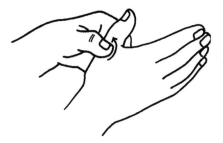

Illustration 2: Press-and-Rotate
Using inside edge of thumb, apply rotating pressure into reflex button.

How to "thumb-walk" across large reflex areas: This technique is often used when working across the hand on a large reflex area such as the liver, lungs, and intestines. With opposite thumb, use very small "steps" across the reflex area. With a tiny range of motion, travel forward, like an inchworm.

This is done by bending your thumb at the first joint, pressing down for a moment, then slightly pulling backward. Move your thumb forward, press down, and pull backward again. Keeping your thumb in contact with flesh, travel across the hand. Then turn the hand around, move your thumb to another reflex trail, and work back across the hand. You will cover a large reflex area if you criss-cross from the outer edge to the inside edge of the hand.

You can also thumb-walk when working up or down a long reflex zone, such as the spinal area, along the thumb side of each hand.

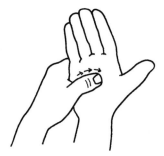

Illustration 3: Thumb-Walk
Slightly bend thumb at first joint, slowly press down, and pull back. Move forward with tiny inchworm steps across reflex area.

How to use the press-and-pull procedure: Bend your thumb at the first joint, and place the working edge on the reflex area. Bend your index finger and place it on the opposite side of the hand. Press into the reflex area simultaneously with your thumb and index finger. Hold for a few seconds, then slide your thumb and finger off the edge of the hand with a slight pinching motion. This stimulates renewed circulation to tight muscles in corresponding zones of the body.

Press-and-pull works especially well along the spinal reflex area on the inside edge of each hand. It also is very effective on the reflex areas of the shoulder and hip, along the outside edges of the hands.

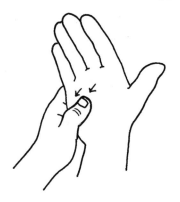

Illustration 4: Press-and-Pull
Place thumb on reflex area, and curve index finger on opposite side of hand. Press together, then slide them concurrently off edge of hand, with a slight pinching motion.

Press-and-Roll Technique: The press-and-roll method works well when working in between the webbing of fingers. Hold the webbing between thumb and index finger (or between thumb and third finger). Press, and slightly roll, your thumb and finger concurrently, over and under the webbing to stimulate healing energy.

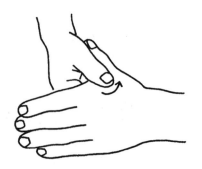

Illustration 5: Press-and-Roll
Hold webbing between thumb and finger. Press-and-roll against both sides of muscle beneath the skin.

How to use the press-and-hold formula: This special technique is often used to calm throbbing pain. It is easy and helps release symptoms of discomfort. Use a firm, steady pressure on a tender reflex point. Or use this method on the end of a zone that corresponds to a painful area in the body. Deep pressure may be uncomfortable when improving irregular health troubles. If pressure is too unpleasant, press-and-hold for a few seconds, let up on pressure, then press-and-hold again. Repeat as needed.

How to Work the Reflexes with Your Fingers

If your thumbs are weak, or tend to tire easily, give them a break: Use finger pressure. Healthy fingers can work freely on reflex areas. It is easy to use one, two, or three fingers at a time. Place a finger on a tender reflex and your thumb on the opposite side of your hand for support. If your thumb hurts, is stiff, or sore, you can rest your hands on your leg, a table, or a firm pillow for support. Your goal is to activate the tender reflexes while you remain in a comfortable position.

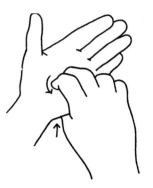

Illustration 6: Press-and-Rotate
With thumb on opposite side of hand for support, use fingers to apply pressure.

Finger press-and-rotate: Apply firm pressure as you slowly rotate your finger on the reflex point. If you need additional pressure on a deep reflex point, you can place your third finger over the second finger for added strength.

The Grip: An effective finger and thumb technique uses the edge of your working index finger. Grip the thumb, or the finger, of opposite hand between your working thumb and finger. Bend your working finger at the first joint, and use the side to press on tender reflex area. Pull bent finger down toward your wrist as you push upward with your thumb. This works well along the edge of both thumbs and all fingers.

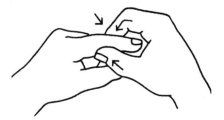

Illustration 7: The Grip
Bend finger at top joint and apply downward pressure. Place thumb on opposite side of leverage.

Finger-walk: Another effective method is to use one, two, or three fingers on the back of the opposite hand. Place fingers side-by-side and "walk" them along each zone. With your fingers on the back of the hand and your thumb on the palm side for support, work with a light pressure, taking very small "steps," press in and slightly pull back. Repeat, gently moving fingers back-and-forth, "walking" them between the metacarpal bones, from fingers to wrist.

Another method is to line fingers together, and walk them sideways up and down the zones. Make several trips to cover all the reflexes on the back of the hand. (See Illustration 9.) This technique can also be used on palms.

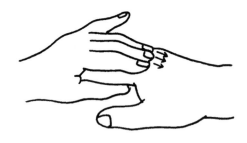

Illustration 8: Finger-Walk
Use two or three fingers to work chest and rib reflex area on back of hands. Make several trips to cover all reflexes on top of each hand.

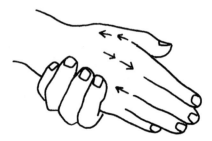

Illustration 9: With thumb on palm, press fingers into reflexes in the back of hand. Work fingers together as a group, or separately up and down each zone.

Give Your Thumbs and Fingers a Rest

If your thumbs fatigue easily, and your fingers feel weak or tired, you can find self-help with the use of a substitute thumb/finger, such as the Magic Reflexer, Reflex Probe, or the Deluxe Hand & Foot Roller. Any of these products can assist you when additional "pressure power" is needed. (See Chapter 5.)

Your goal is to work tenderness out of the reflex points, stimulating internal energies to help readjust health imperfections and improve physical and mental well-being. Your intent is to create happiness and good health for yourself and those you care about.

Hand, Finger, and Thumb Rotations

Hand rotations: Rotating the hands will help awaken nerves and stimulate circulation. Gently rotate at wrist in small circles, then medium circles, and then make circles as large as you can. Move your hands clockwise a few times, then counterclockwise a few times. This will encourage the movement of lymph, which will help defend the body against disease.

If hands are stiff or tight, do not force them to move, just gently wave them in one direction, and then in another direction. These movements are helpful for improving flexibility as well as warming the hands and balancing the body's energies.

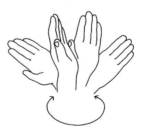

Illustration 10: Rotate each hand to the left; then to the right. This will stimulate renewed lymph and blood flow.

Finger and thumb rotations: If fingers and thumbs are rigid or inflexible, you can awaken stimulation within them by gently rocking each finger back and forth between your thumb and two fingers of the opposite hand. Repeat over each joint, using mild pressure and traction.

Gently rotate each finger in tiny circles, first clockwise, then counterclockwise to relax tension and loosen joints. If this feels good, increase the size of circles. If it hurts, do not force your fingers to move.

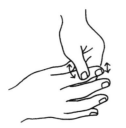

Illustration 11: Gently twist and rock each finger to release tautness in joints.

If fingers are too sore or stiff to move individually, try moving them all at once. Move them up and down, as if you are waving to someone across the room. Then turn your hand sideways and move fingers back and forth like a fish tail.

Be careful: Do not force fingers to move, especially after surgery or in the case of a healing fracture or inflammation. Use common sense; if fingers are not flexible, it is dangerous to force them to move.

REFLEX WITH CAUTION THE FIRST WEEK

The first week you use reflexology, pressure should not be applied for more than a few seconds on any one point. If reflexes are over-stimulated, the body will have a lot of toxins to dispel all at once. This can make a person feel indisposed for a few hours after the workout.

To prevent the ill feelings, drink a glass of water before and after your reflex workout. This will help your body flush out and release the excess materials. Therefore remember, whether using your fingers or a self-help reflex tool, give a very short workout the first week.

Once the body flushes out digested metabolic waste, nature's own energetic power centers will start correcting and balancing the internal systems. This will allow the body to revitalize, renew, and repair itself naturally. These are the miracles your wonderful body can perform with the simple help of reflexology.

How Much Pressure Should Be Used

Always use a gentle touch, yet place enough pressure on the reflex point to stimulate renewed circulation. Use from one ounce to six pounds of pressure on a reflex point in the hands. The one-ounce pressure would be used on an *extremely* sore spot. The six-pound pressure would be on a very deep reflex, or in an area with very thick skin. (To check this amount of pressure, place your thumb, or fingers, on a produce scale at your local market.)

The more you work the reflexes, the better you will be able to judge the pressure. Your intuition will help you decide the correct touch for an effective performance.

You will not want to put very much pressure on the elderly, children, pregnant women, or chronically ill people; a very tender, loving touch is recommended for them. They will each require special care and kindhearted contact. Always be sensitive to, and thoughtful of, their individual needs.

How Long Should Pressure Be Applied

When you work a reflex button, you need to give it medium pressure for about seven seconds. If this button is sore, it is telling you that the corresponding body part is weak or in trouble. When a gland is not functioning properly, it will respond to the stimulus.

A short-term, rotating motion on a reflex is enough to send electrical information to the coinciding sick gland, and the energy around it increases the healing action. Work the reflex at least every other day while trying to stimulate a certain malfunctioning gland from congestion. It takes only seconds for the stimuli to travel from the reflex point to the connecting organ or gland—about the time it takes a lightbulb to start warming after turning it on.

So you see, it is within your power to strengthen the body and sharpen the mind. As the saying goes, "Today is the first day of the rest of your life," so make it count. Just reach out your hands, and use reflexology on all the necessary reflex buttons. In a short period of time, you will have control of your health and be able to thoroughly enjoy your future!

How to Know Which Reflex Buttons to Press

Follow the guide set for you in Chapter 4. The best reflex session is a complete workout to both hands. Work across all divisions, as well as up and down all five zones on *both hands* to encourage a flow of healing energy throughout the whole body.

Work a little longer on the sore spots, but if it hurts too much, move on to another reflex button and then return to the sore spot later on. Remember our motto: "If it hurts, work it out!" But not in one day. Eventually you will notice that you have "worked out" all the tenderness from the reflex points in your hands. When you no longer feel soreness in the reflexes, celebrate, as this is nature's way of telling you there is no longer any trouble within the corresponding body parts.

PRACTICE MAKES PERFECT

It may take a little practice to catch on to the most effective method, and the most convenient and comfortable for you. Your health is truly in your wonderful hands if you will take time to turn the Magic Key of Reflexology as given in this book.

Learning to Work the Reflex Points in Your Fingers and Hands

You have studied the charts and basic techniques, and now you have a general idea of how each part of your body has a corresponding reflex located in the hands and fingers. In explaining how to work the various reflex points and their coinciding areas in the body, we'll follow the Hand Charts B and C (pages 11 and 12).

We will start with the top of the thumb and fingers, and work the reflexes corresponding to the head. Then we will progress to the rest of the hands, explaining the reflexes and body areas as we go. See Charts A and B (pages 10 and 11), and refer to the Zone Chart (page 14) as guidelines throughout this chapter.

HOW TO WORK REFLEXES IN THUMBS AND FINGERS

As explained earlier, reflexes in the thumb correspond to certain areas of the head; the left thumb and fingers stimulate the left side of the head, and the right thumb and fingers, the right side of the head. You

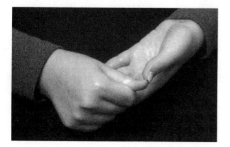

Photo 3: Stimulate healing energy to the brain and sinuses by applying direct pressure on top of each thumb. Repeat on the top of each finger on both hands.

will find that the fingers are very significant, as they particularly seem to control the nerves and mentality.

Start with upper end of thumb: Begin the reflex work by rolling your right fingernail across the top of the left thumb at its very tip (see Photo 3, page 30). If it's easier for you, you can apply pressure with the top of your opposite thumb, or use a reflex tool. Be careful not to bruise the flesh under the nail itself.

Next, take the palm side of your left thumb between the right thumb and index finger, and drop down to the pad that is located above the first joint. (See Photo 51, page 280) Press deeply into it with the edge of your right thumb. As you will notice on the charts, this is the reflex to the pituitary and hypothalamus glands in the brain. Because of its close proximity, you will also be working the reflex to the pineal gland. Stimulation of the pituitary gland often means a new lease on life for young and old.

These are very important endocrine glands located deep in the brain. Therefore, the reflexes in the thumb are also deep. You may get better results by using a self-help reflex tool, such as the Probe, shown in Photo 4, or any blunt instrument that will help press more firmly into the reflex buttons. Be sure to cover the whole pad with a pressing, rolling motion.

Now work the edge of your thumb, and on around to the back (or topside) of the thumb just below the nail. Work this whole area down to the base of the thumb, searching thoroughly for tender reflexes as you go.

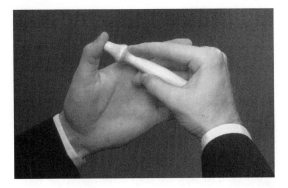

Photo 4: Working the deep reflexes of the pituitary, hypothalamus, and pineal gland, with the help of a Reflex Probe.

Working reflexes at the base of the thumb: Just above where the thumb joins the hand, we find reflexes to the throat, neck, tonsils, thyroid, and vocal cord. Press your right thumb into the reflex of the thyroid gland, at the base of the left thumb. You will work all along this area. To reach the parathyroid you will press a little deeper.

As you will notice on Chart B, page 11, there are many reflexes at the base of the thumb; do not neglect any section of the thumb, no matter how small or insignificant it may appear to you. Only by reaching all the reflexes will you get the full benefits of reflexology.

Repeat the reflex work on the right thumb in the same manner. By this time you should actually feel your body responding and renewing its vital forces, and notice the muscles in your neck are relaxing as if by magic.

How reflexology stopped a stiff neck: A retired friend who had the habit of falling asleep while reading invariably woke up with a stiff neck due to faulty posture. She quickly learned from me how to work the stiffness out of her neck, by working the reflexes in her thumbs, to obtain immediate relief.

Working reflexes in the fingers: Now let us go over the fingers which, as the charts indicate, hold the reflexes to the nerves and sinuses. One of the best ways to work sinus reflexes is in the tips of the fingers. Roll the thumbnail back and forth over each finger just at the edge of the nail, as you did on the thumb (see Photo 3, page 29). When you do this correctly, you will usually feel a tender prickling sensation as if you are pressing on splinters in the tips of your fingers. Roll the right thumb over the tips of the left fingers and use the left thumb to roll along the tips of the right fingers.

Since the sinuses affect several areas in the head, you can readily see how working the reflexes in the fingers to corresponding zones will benefit sinus conditions.

Now let us concentrate on our fingers for a few minutes. Work over them slowly and completely to stimulate renewed energy through each zone. Work all around the finger, by pressing on the *back and front* of it (see Photo 5, page 32). When you get to the webbing between the fingers, pinch and massage it well, as this will benefit your eyes, ears, and sinuses. When you do find a tender spot, work on it a few seconds, then go on to the next finger.

Continue your work on the sides of each finger; here we find the reflexes to the nerves. Work *both sides* of each finger (see Photo 6,

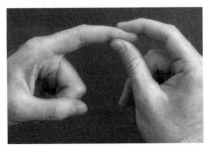

Photo 5: Position for applying pressure to the anterior and posterior (front and back) of the fingers.

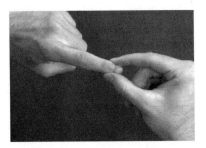

Photo 6: Position for applying lateral pressure on both sides of the fingers.

page 32), searching for tender spots as you work down toward the hand, as you did with the thumb.

Keep working up and down each finger, pressing and rolling deep enough so that you can feel the three-dimensional firmness of the muscle and bone underneath. The nerve reflexes at the end of each zone, as well as along the side of each finger, may be used to bring about an anesthetic effect, to decrease pain without drugs.

Be sure to work both thumbs and all fingers on both hands, so that forceful life pulsations may be manifested into all of the glandular regions of your body.

HOW TO WORK BETWEEN THE WEBBING OF FINGERS

The webbing between fingers has many important reflexes, several of which are "assistants" to other reflex areas, such as the neck, sinuses, eyes, ears, and all sensory organs. You will work these reflex areas by placing the first finger and thumb of the opposite hand over and under the webbing. With a pinching, rolling technique, gently work the reflex points next to the small muscles, and up against the bones underneath the skin. Work between all fingers. You will be surprised at the tender spots you find here.

The webbing between the thumb and index finger: The webbing here is much larger than the others, and we find that the reflexes in it correspond to a larger area of the body. (See Chart C, page 12.) This is also a pain-control reflex button that can be stimulated by pressure. Steady pressure can cause a release of natural pain-inhibiting chemicals called "endorphins." Because there are some very miraculous and powerful reflex buttons here in this V-shaped part of the hand, we give this reflex area a special name for reference throughout this book: we call it the "Magical V."

To work this powerful section of your hand, spread your thumb and index finger. With opposite thumb and index finger, gently press and work the webbing thoroughly, from the thin part back into the thicker muscle area. Now change hands using the same pinch and roll technique. Work the Magical V on your opposite hand, being sure to cover the whole area (see Illustration 12, page 34).

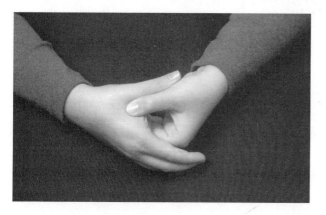

Photo 7: Position for working reflexes in the "Magical V" section of the right hand.

The benefits of working this area: We find reflexes not only to the throat and neck, but also to the thyroid, stomach, and other internal organs. For instance, by working the correct spot, you can help relieve a swollen throat, sinus problems, allergies, hay fever, asthma, coughing, fainting, dizziness, arthritis pain, indigestion, constipation, headaches, toothaches, labor pain, hot flashes, anxiety, depression, nausea, and hangovers.

Moreover, healing energy can be stimulated through various muscles that pull on the spine by working the Magical V along the side of your index finger (see Photo 25 in Chapter 20). You will learn additional specific points to work throughout the following chapters.

Finding the correct reflex location: Note in Illustration 12 that the connecting metacarpal bone is at the end of the V, almost to the wrist. Within this section of the hand is a network of muscles and nerves. There is also a cluster of reflex points here.

You can position your thumb and the index finger (or third finger) of opposite hand, above and below the Magical V. Exert pressure on the webbing or up against the basal joints, with a press-and-rotate movement. This is a special combination of reflex points. Several buttons within the V correspond to different functions of the body. For instance, here are a few samples:

1. Apply pressure up against thumb to stop frontal headaches.
2. Direct pressure toward the index finger to ease a cold.
3. Work within the center section to stop indigestion and stomachaches.
4. Place pressure on the back of the hand, at the deepest point of the Magical V, to stop cramps and hot flashes.

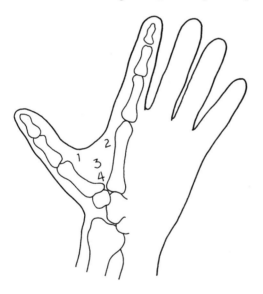

Illustration 12: There are several reflex points within the Magical V. These special buttons are often called "pain eliminators."

It will be easy to find the reflex button you are looking for once you study the charts. In many cases, it is more effective to stop pain by merely holding a steady pressure on a certain reflex, instead of using a pressing, rolling motion. When you find a sore spot, press firmly for two minutes or longer and take several slow deep breaths to relieve distress.

EASY TECHNIQUES FOR FINDING REFLEX POINTS IN YOUR PALMS

You know how to find all the reflex buttons in your fingers and those in the webbing between them. Now let's look at those in the hands, and check out their connections to other areas of the body.

Let us first look at the hand charts. You will notice at the base of the fingers that it says "ears" and "eyes." With your right thumb, press on the pad just about where the fingers join your left hand. Use a press-and-roll motion here as you search out tender spots. When you find a sore spot, keep working it for a few seconds to release a flow of electrical life force into the congested area, thus giving nature a helping hand in healing whatever the malfunction might be.

This will be true in all cases where you find a tender spot on any reflex. Our therapy motto is "if a reflex hurts, rub it out." Any sore spot on a reflex indicates malfunctioning in the corresponding part of the body, no matter how remote it may be from the reflex button being stimulated.

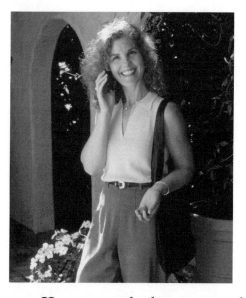

Photo 8: Stimulating reflexes in the left hand (shown here with a Magic Reflexer) sends currents of healing energy through the left side of the body.

How to work the upper pads: Next, you will work the reflexes to the lungs and bronchial tubes, which are located on the upper pads of your hands. With the thumb of your right hand, work along this whole area. It may be easier for you to work both hands as we move along. Don't ever give yourself only half a workout by over-looking one of your hands. You can see on your charts how this would stimulate only one side of your body and neglect some of the glands and organs on the untreated side.

Working the upper pad on the left hand also sends healing circulation to the heart and circulatory system, which is a large area. You will also be working the bronchial reflexes, as they are all interrelated. Work the upper pad on the left palm as well as the upper part on the back of the left hand. Work completely across from the inside to the outside of the hand.

Work reflexes across the middle of hands: Let us move on to the stomach reflexes which, as you can see on your chart, are located in the soft area just under the thumb of both hands and across the hand a bit. (Refer to Photo 26, page 151.) When you work the reflexes to the stomach, you will also be sending vital energy to the pancreas, duodenum, kidneys, and adrenals, because these organs overlap each other. You will work this area with the thumb of the opposite hand using the press-and-rotate motion.

Now let us progress to the center of the palm. The solar plexus reflex area is located near the stomach, and the diaphragm reflex runs across both hands, just under the lung reflexes.

Since our body is three dimensional, many organs and glands unite in this area and work together to help maintain us. This is where we run into congestion of the reflexes and it will be almost impossible to work one without sending some currents of vital life forces surging through other close-lying glands and organs. This is why we can never take our bodies for granted. There are many wonderful functions taking place, hidden beneath our skin.

Next, we find the reflexes to the adrenal and the kidney located in zone two of the hand (see Zone Chart, page 14, and Photo 33, page 204). Notice how the thumb is held in position to work these two reflexes.

You will notice on the right hand that by moving the thumb over onto the pad under the little finger, you will be on the outside edge of the reflex to the liver. (See Photo 35, page 213.) Use a criss-cross technique to cover the entire reflex area. Moving down a bit and about half-way across the hand, you will find the reflex to the gall bladder.

Working across the lower section of each hand, you will be on the colon reflex. Moving toward the wrist are the reflexes to the small intestines and bladder. The appendix is on the right hand only, as we have only one appendix, and it is on the right side of the body.

If self-help tools other than the fingers are used, such as the Magic Reflexer or the Deluxe Hand & Foot Roller, forceful life pulsations will be manifested in all of these regions at once, instead of just one at a time. Therefore, the use of reflex tools is often helpful in the case of constipation and other digestive or intestinal problems.

HOW TO WORK REFLEXES ON BACK (OR TOP) OF HANDS

Refer to Chart C (page 12) and notice the reflex areas on the back of each hand. The skin is thinner here and reflexes are not so sensitive. Therefore, most reflex work will be done on the palms of the hands. However, working the Magical V on the back of each hand is very effective.

Work reflexes on the back of each hand to send healing energy to chest, breast, ribs, lungs, the circulatory system, and muscles. Working the backs of hands can be done with the fingers, or thumb, of the opposite hand. (See Illustrations 8 and 9 on page 24.)

Now, let us look at the reflexes to the lower lumbar spine and sex glands. As you can see by looking at your charts, they are located mostly on the wrist. (Refer to Chapter 32 on sex glands.) Use a press-and-rotate motion or the press-and-pull method to work these reflexes.

The importance of the lymph glands: While we are still on the wrist, turn the hand over and on the back of the wrist, you will find the reflexes to the lymph glands. Use thumb or fingers to work across the back of the wrist several times as the lymph glands can always use a little natural help in their work of taking care of any infections that might invade the body.

Some Reflex Buttons May Be Difficult to Locate

Because we use our hands all day long, the hand and finger reflex buttons may not be so sensitive, or so easy to locate, as those in the feet. Toes and feet are very receptive to reflexology. This is because they are usually well protected by shoes, socks, or slippers. When we do go barefoot, we walk on soft surfaces such as rugs and lawns, which keep our feet tender. Therefore the reflex points are easy to find.

Searching for sore spots in the hands and fingers can be a challenge at times. For this reason, I will explain the use of several beneficial self-help tools which will enable you to work the reflexes in your hands more thoroughly. (See Chapter 5.)

Nature's Gift to Relieve Pain

We do not claim that reflexology is a panacea for every ailment, but neither is any other method. Nature has given us a marvelous gift with which we can relieve pain and suffering and bring renewed health to the body, and we should make use of it in every way possible. In reflexology we find a safe natural way to health, and the techniques are so simple and harmless they can be used by anyone.

Evangelist of Oral Roberts Treated by Dr. Fitzgerald

Dear Mrs. Carter:

It really made me feel good to read your letter and to know that you too were a Christian. You wound up your letter by saying "May God continue to bless you." I am 82 years old and still going strong. A Trustee of Oral Roberts Evang. Association and his University, and an International Director of the Full Gospel Business Men's Fellowship International.

I knew Dr. Fitzgerald of Hartford, Connecticut. He was one of the most patient men I ever knew. He knew that he had made a discovery (Zone Therapy) and took a lot of time to work it out.

I remember many years ago I had to have an operation on an Inguinal Hernia and I wanted to try out Zone Therapy. The only anesthetic I had was a little novocaine in my side. I applied pressure on the very ends of my fingers on the operating table. And while the operation was not absolutely painless, I was able to stand it. The novocaine was most ineffective. I also remember that I had some pain elsewhere. I do not remember where. I could not find the pressure zone as he called it at the time. He said, "Look in the web between the third and fourth fingers," and sure enough there it was. I could hardly touch it. And it was the same between the corresponding toes. I am a D.D.S., Past President of Hartford Dental Society, Conn. State Dental Assoc., and also N. England Dental Society. With Kindest Regards and I know God will Bless you, too. In His wonderful and powerful Name.

Dr. J. F. Barton

CHAPTER 5

How to Use Self-Help Tools at Home to Relieve Pain

When Dr. Fitzgerald first started using pressure on the reflexes to alleviate pain and cure many diseases, he discovered how to make use of several tools found around the house. These tools helped him hold a steady pressure on zones for a prolonged period of time in order to anesthetize certain parts of the body. He used them to ease toothache pain, earaches, labor pains, and many other painful ailments.

By putting pressure on the tips of certain fingers and holding it a few minutes, he found that he could effectively ease pain in the corresponding part of the body. To save time, he found that ordinary clothespins would work better than his fingers, and it was a lot less tiring. He discovered that with special tools he could also have his patients keep up the treatments at home, using simple, ingenious little implements.

The doctor also found that the teeth of a hard comb worked best in many situations. The comb could be used to hold pressure on several reflex points at a time, not only on the fingers, but on all parts of the hands—and this simple method could be used safely at home when needed.

Small rubber balls were used to improve hand strength and speed recovery to those who were weak. These therapeutic balls are still being used today by many doctors and in hospitals to boost energy and renew circulation for patients with arthritis. They are also helpful rehabilitative tools for stroke victims and those with various other kinds of paralysis.

In this book, you will see illustrations and directions on the use of several improved self-help reflex tools that have been designed especially for reflexology. These may be obtained at your local bookstore, health store, or from Stirling Enterprises, whose telephone number is on page 291.

It is not essential that you have these reflex tools to obtain beneficial and lasting results when doing your reflex work. Reflexology is a natural way to health, and the natural use of your fingers will work wonders in releasing the universal flow of vital life forces. This healing dynamism sends energy surging through all the channels of your body, bringing you a renewed state of health and vitality. You will be given directions on how to use reflexology with the fingers, as well as with some of the self-help tools, in the following chapters.

HOW TO USE THE MAGIC REFLEXER

In my search for a simple tool that would sufficiently work most of the reflexes in the hands, I developed the Magic Reflexer, shown in Photo 9.

Therapeutic treatment with a rubber ball has been used by doctors and in hospitals for years. Patients who have arthritis in the fingers, hands, and arms have been given a small rubber ball to hold, and told to squeeze it as much as they could, with satisfying results.

I felt there was a need for a self-help tool that would press in and stimulate the reflexes in the hands for even better results. Therefore, I designed a new type of ball with small, but sturdy fingertips on it for this purpose. The beneficial results have been even more than I had hoped for.

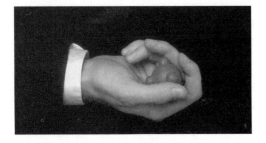

Photo 9: How to hold the Magic Reflexer in your hand. Notice how the little massaging fingers are defined so they can press in and work the reflex points with gratifying results.

Case History of First Experiment with Magic Reflexer

When I got my first sample Magic Reflexer, I gave it to my husband to try on our way home. He really liked the feel of it, and kept squeezing and rolling it in one hand and then the other as we drove home. Suddenly he said, "I feel kind of sick." I told him to quit using the reflexer which he did, and the sick feeling stopped. *He had over-massaged the reflexes in his hands.* This is when we realized how powerful this little massager is!

Magic Reflexer Relieves Aching Arm

My son-in-law was having trouble with his arm going to sleep at night, and aching at times during the day. He tried using the Magic Reflexer every night as directed, for about two weeks, and has had no more trouble with his arm since. He still uses it daily to make sure the trouble does not return.

Techniques for Using the Magic Reflexer

Take the Magic Reflexer in one hand and close your fingers around it. Now squeeze. Notice how its small, yet strong "fingers" press into several reflexes of your hand at one time. Roll it over and it will press into a different set of reflexes. Each time you roll it a little, it reaches different reflex points (see Photos 10a and 10b on page 42).

Do this for about two minutes, then change to the other hand, again working it around for about two minutes. You will immediately feel a stimulation of magnetic vitality surging through your whole body. You will not want to lay this little Magic Reflexer down. But remember: *Don't over-work the reflexes!* You can use it again tomorrow or maybe later in the day if you feel okay after using it the first time.

By looking at Chart B (page 11) you can see that the reflexes are crowded into a small area. Notice in Chart A (page 10) how most of the organs and glands on both sides of the body will be stimulated into renewed life as many of the reflex buttons are pressed. You can easily see why this little reflexer works such magic when used as directed. The Magic Reflexer is revitalizing almost the whole body.

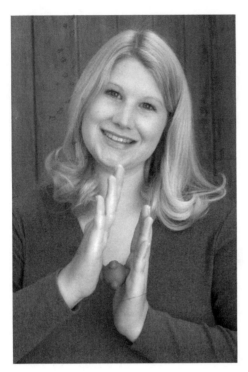

Photo 10a: Roll the Magic Reflexer between both hands for a double force of healing stimulation.

How to get double benefits from the Magic Reflexer: Take the reflexer and place it in the palm of your hand. Now cup the other hand over it, clasping your fingers around each other. Roll the reflexer between the hands in several directions. Feel how the little "fingers" press into the reflex buttons of both hands simultaneously.

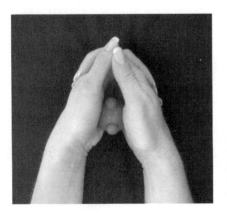

Photo 10b: Interlace fingers and place the reflexer between palms, and press-and-roll in several directions.

Using the Magic Reflexer on fingers and thumbs: Take up the Magic Reflexer and start pressing one of its small fingers into the end of your thumb. Next press one of the "little fingers" along the sides of each thumb, pressing and rolling all the way to the base of your thumb. Repeat this rolling-pressing motion on each of the other fingers.

You will be surprised at the sore spots this little magic ball will find for you, in the fingers as well as in the hands. Remember our motto, "If it is sore, work it out." However, don't try to do it the first day or even the first week. Although reflexology does seem to work miracles in many cases, take your time. Your body was a long time getting into the condition it is now in, so don't try to shock it into perfect working order in just a few days. Give it a chance to rebuild into perfection.

Athletes Love the Magic Reflexer

I talk with many athletes who have developed strength and endurance by using the Magic Reflexer. They enjoy using it before and after their favorite sports activity. The squeezing motion helps develop neglected muscles. It immensely helps the overall development professional athletes need in their fingers, hands, wrists, and forearms. These developed muscles also help prevent future injury from a strenuous game, or soreness from overdoing everyday activities.

Golfers find that by rolling it around in their hands several times a day, they improve the flexibility and control needed to swing the club accurately. It also leaves a feeling of relaxation and confidence when used just before a game.

Bowlers find the Magic Reflexer helps keep their fingers, hands, wrists, and forearms strong, yet limber enough for a good game. It is very relaxing to use after the game is over, too.

The younger generation loves the Magic Reflexer, as it is a popular pre-game exercise used before their competitive adventures such as badminton, baseball, basketball, and tennis.

My teenage grandson Kevin used it to strengthen his fingers and hands before an archery tournament. He took first place in his age group.

One young woman took the Magic Reflexer from her locker before a volleyball game, used it in each hand for a few minutes, and then tossed it to a teammate so she could use it, too. They told me, "It's fun and easy to use, we feel it builds up our wrist muscles, and strengthens our fingers for better grip, and gives us the extra control we need to win. And the reflex stimulation that goes into our body can help us hit with more power!"

Several young men and women are now taking the Magic Reflexer along with them wherever they go. They are carrying the reflexers in their backpack, purse, or briefcase and use them when needed to stimulate circulation, relieve ill complaints, or just to exercise for joint and muscle power. They find them great to share with friends, too!

How the Magic Reflexer Strengthened an Artist's Hands

A very popular artist whom I knew was devoting his full time to painting pictures, murals in churches, and also teaching art. I noticed that he had started dropping his brush quite frequently during art classes. One day I stayed and after everyone had left I asked him about it. A worried look came over his face and he said, "I don't know what is wrong. I just suddenly lose control of my right hand, for no reason that I know of. If I lose the use of my hand I am done. I have devoted my life to the study of art, and this is all I can do and it is the work I love."

I took one of the Magic Reflexers out of my purse and showed it to him. I asked if he would try it for a while and see what it would do for him. Since he knew that I was a reflexologist and had much success with so many cases, he was delighted to take my advice and try the reflexer.

I told him to work it in both hands and especially the right hand every time he got a chance. The next week, when I went to class, I noticed he didn't drop his brush once.

Later, he told me how grateful he was for such a simple remedy, which he claims saved not only his business, but his happiness. It also alleviated some malfunctioning in his body which might have proved serious if it hadn't been stopped. We never did know what had caused the trouble, but were more than delighted that it had vanished. This occurred several years ago and, thus far, there has been no recurrence of his trouble and he has been able to go on to even greater works of art. He says, "Thanks to the little Magic Reflexer," which he still uses every day.

HOW TO STOP PAIN WITH A REFLEX COMB AND REFLEX CLAMPS

When a steady pressure is held for a short period of time on a reflex, it can cause an anesthetic effect in the corresponding part of the body.

If we hold pressure on reflexes in the thumb or the ends of certain fingers for a few minutes, pain in the corresponding zone will numb, often eliminating the cause of discomfort.

The Advantage of Using Reflex Clamps

You can apply steady pressure with your own thumb and finger, using the opposite hand, or you can use a Reflex Clamp. Pressure should be held from two to fifteen minutes at a time.

Early in the nineteenth century, before the reflex clamps were designed, some doctors used rubber bands to hold pressure on the reflexes for an anesthetic effect. Now many use their fingers, or clamps. The reflex clamps are a lot safer and easier to use. They are designed to give an anesthetic effect, without interfering with the circulation.

When pressure is placed on a zone, it helps stop pain within the corresponding body part. We can see how this would enfold all body parts functioning within that zone from head to toe. (See Chart E on page 14.) When waves of tension and pain are reduced, blood and oxygen supply improves. This allows the nerves to function better, and the body is able to reestablish harmony and balance, which lets it mend and rebuild itself.

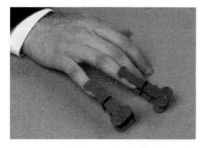

Photo 11: Use Reflex Clamps on fourth and fifth fingers to help anesthetize pain within zones 4 and 5.

Look at Photo 11 and see how reflex clamps are fastened on the fourth and fifth fingers. Some cases of complete deafness have been reversed, with nothing more than this simple pressure on the end of the third, fourth, and fifth fingers several times a day. Many people have been able to hear better within a few minutes after the clamps have been placed on their fingers. You will read in Chapter 8 almost unbelievable cases of the deaf regaining their hearing in this way.

Reflex clamps are safe and easy to use for quick relief from many types of pain. By looking at chart D, you can visualize how clamps placed on certain fingers of the right hand will affect the right side of the body, and when placed on the left hand, the left side of the body will receive the benefit.

Doctor Demonstrates Proof of Reflexology

Dr. White tells of cases where he used pressure on the fingers with good results. "By placing pressure on a fellow doctor's thumb and index finger on his right hand, I was able to anesthetize part of the right side of his face. The same day in a hotel, I met a woman who had a severe headache. I exerted pressure upon the fingers in the indicated zones and within five minutes, the headache had disappeared. I had the same success in treating a toothache."

How to Benefit from Using Reflex Combs

Pressing and working the reflexes in the hands with fingers will give satisfactory results most of the time, but there will be certain cases where a steady pressure will be needed for several minutes at a time. This is where the value of using the comb technique comes in.

Any type of comb may be used in an emergency, but keep in mind that most combs are made of plastic and could very easily break and injure the hands or fingers if too much pressure were placed on them. The doctors recommended that a special strong comb be used in zone therapy for this reason.

How reflex combs help renew stimulation: Reflex combs are self-help tools that must be used very gently. They can reach several reflex points, and are effective in stimulating renewed circulation. The teeth of this sturdy reflex comb can be used to press into the tips of the fingers (see Photo 61, page 285). When pressing your thumb pad on the end of a reflex comb, you are activating energy to your brain. Here you will find reflex buttons that correspond to three very important endocrine glands in the head: the pituitary, hypothalamus, and pineal.

Using the reflex comb to locate sore spots: Gently press the teeth of the comb into the palm of your hand. Press it into different areas, holding it in each position for a few seconds to get the feel of it. When you find sore spots, hold it a few seconds. If you find the reflexes are too tender, then use the back of the comb for a few days.

Using this method, it is easy to search for tender reflex areas that are warning you of trouble spots in your body. Refer to your charts to see which areas in the body are sending out distress signals. Remember to work the reflexes on *both* hands.

HOW TO REGAIN HEALTH WITH THE DELUXE HAND & FOOT ROLLER

The most popular self-help reflex tool on the market is the Deluxe Hand & Foot Roller. It has many benefits, and is great for renewing circulation of both blood and lymph, which is an important part of enhancing general health. This special roller is used for improving energy flow as well as for encouraging general relaxation.

Easy to use: First, get into a comfortable position, then place your hands around the reflex roller. Slowly press and squeeze your hands on all sides of it to stimulate reflexes and encourage circulation (see Photo 12a, page 48). Next, place your thumb on a large nodule, or "massaging-finger," of the roller (see Photo 12b, page 48). Rock and roll your thumb back and forth, searching for sore spots. When you find a tender reflex point, work on it for a few seconds and then move on.

Another method is to place the deluxe roller between your palms and move your hands back and forth, moving the roller between them. (See Photo 12c.) If done slowly, this is a wonderful, relaxing treat for your whole body. As the little "fingers" on the roller press into your palms, you can feel the tension draining from the tight muscles of your body.

If you feel tired and want more vim and vigor, use quick movements to invigorate circulation throughout the reflex zones. To do this, roll your hands back and forth quickly against the roller "fingers." This renews vital currents of energy to effectively increase your stamina and supercharge your vitality.

This deluxe roller feels great against the feet, too. Simply place it on the floor and roll it back and forth under each foot for an extraordinary feeling of renewed liveliness.

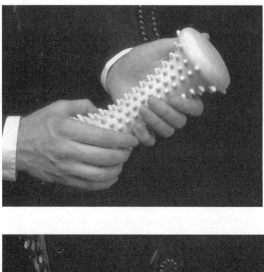

Photo 12a: Pressing each hand against the "massaging-fingers" of the Deluxe Roller will stimulate reflexes.

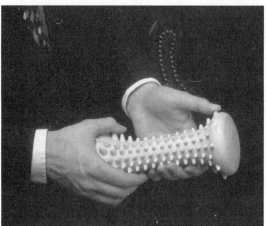

Photo 12b: Simply press one finger at a time to work specific reflex points.

If your joints are stiff or your hands are weak: You will benefit from using a self-help tool, such as this one, to assist you in reaching the healing zones. You can place the roller on a table or counter top, and gently roll it under each hand for one minute (see Photo 43, page 254). Press down with one hand over the top of the other if you need additional pressure. This way you will be sure that the roller "fingers" work the reflex points. Reverse hands and repeat.

Portable and easy to use anytime: I know many professional workers who have Deluxe Rollers in their desk drawers. When they need a reflex break, to either reduce stress or increase their stamina,

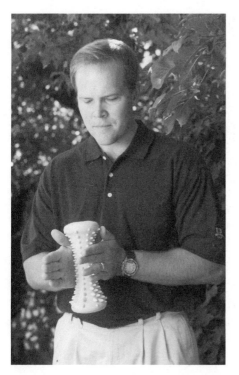

Photo 12c: Moving the Deluxe Hand & Foot Roller back-and-forth between palms will encourage renewed circulation.

they roll it between their hands, or take off their shoes and work the roller under their feet.

Several have mentioned that the roller really has saved their day. It energizes the healing forces within the body, and gets rid of such suffering as cramps, headaches, and stomachaches.

When all the energy zones are stimulated at one time, it gives your body currents of invigorating new circulation. Why shouldn't you feel a renewed exhilaration of energy almost instantly? This is instant vitality at your fingertips!

The knowledge of reflexology will open a whole new way of life, not only for you, but also for others whom you will be able to free from the darkness of illness and pain. The self-help method of reflexology has been used for many years to control suffering and discomfort.

So do not hesitate to use self-help reflex tools if they will benefit your state of health in any way. Take advantage of this proven, revolutionary approach to health management. Reflexology is safe and natural; you can use it without leaving home or your place of work; and most important, without drugs or harsh medications.

REFLEXOLOGY IS A GODSEND

I do not advise anyone to depend on reflexology as a cure-all. Nevertheless, if this simple, harmless method of applying pressure to certain areas of the body, hands and feet, and fingers and toes will alleviate pain from any cause, it is a godsend for the whole human race.

The acupuncture doctors are using the same principles of stimulating this life force to anesthetize pain and heal diseases by using needles, which we know can be quite dangerous if used by the layman or even an untrained practitioner. We can be thankful that our doctors rediscovered the western style of reflexology by using the simple pressure method of the fingers and other harmless tools that we can keep in our homes to accomplish like results.

CHAPTER 6

Your Life and Your Endocrine Glands

Let us give our attention to the all-important endocrine glands. These glands are scattered in various places throughout the body, and are all interrelated, as they supplement and depend on each other. They secrete hormones directly into the bloodstream; these messengers control the pace at which certain organs or glands work.

All together, the body manufactures over a hundred chemical messengers called hormones. The digestive system makes several hormones, the ovaries at least six different estrogens, the glands in the brain produce about twenty various hormones, and the adrenals secrete over thirty steroid hormones. In this chapter, we are going to name only a few of the best-known hormones that the endocrine glands produce.

In conjunction with the nervous system, the endocrine glands direct and coordinate all of the body's activities. Their normal functions and development are of great importance to the well-being of every individual. (See the Endocrine Gland Chart on page 57).

I am including this chapter on the endocrine gland system because of its influence, not only on your health, but also on your looks, your happiness, and your way of life.

THREE IMPORTANT GLANDS ARE LOCATED IN THE BRAIN

Hypothalamus: This gland sits atop the control center in the brain and is attached to the pituitary by a short stem. It instructs the pituitary to release hormones to certain target glands.

The reflex to this gland is in the pad of each thumb. When you work the reflex to the pituitary gland, you will also be working the reflex to the hypothalamus gland. They work together to coordinate various activities of the nervous system and regulate how much hormone the other glands secrete.

Pituitary: This gland takes some directions from the hypothalamus, but it is the commander of the whole army of endocrine glands, and is often called the "king" gland. The front part secretes several hormones. Most of them act as dispatch riders, carrying commands to the body's other ductless glands. One of these hormones is the growth hormone, which determines whether you grow into a giant or develop into a smaller person.

The back of this gland holds hormones for the hypothalamus, which controls the concentration of urine and contractions during labor.

When this gland is functioning in perfect order, growth will be normal. If you have a child who is not developing as you think he should, give nature a chance to normalize the function of this gland by stimulating the reflex to the pituitary. This may help give your child a chance to develop a normal stature.

Working the reflex in the center pad of both thumbs (and also the big toes) will bring the necessary stimulation to this gland. If it hurts, then it is surely calling for help by sending you a message that there is trouble with the commander.

Pineal: This is a very small pine-cone-shaped gland. It responds indirectly to the amount of light that our eyes reflect to it. When it gets dark, the pineal gland switches on and begins secreting the hormone *melatonin* that helps our body sleep. When we see light, the production of this hormone stops. It signals the body when it is time to go to sleep and when it is time to wake up.

A famous philosopher from France, René Descartes, once wrote, "The pineal gland is the place where mind and body meet." Eons ago, in the long story of evolution, it was a sort of primitive eye in many animals.

In its present position inside the human brain, it acts within the body as a kind of organizer or harmonizer, controlling the development of the glands and keeping their functions in proper

balance. It controls the daily rhythms of our lives and notifies the adolescent body when to start maturing by sending out hormones when a child is between 9 and 13 years old. It also secretes a hormone to regulate menstrual cycles.

A pathological condition of this gland strongly influences the sex glands, causing premature development of the whole system. The endocrine system is kept harmonious and effective by the normal activity of the pineal gland.

The reflexes to this gland are also located in the thumb pad (and big toe), just a little toward the inside of each thumb. Remember to work both hands. Also, work the reflex areas on top of each finger, as each one represents a zone, through which energy travels to the brain. (See Chart D, page 13.)

HOW TO ACTIVATE MORE HORMONE-PRODUCING GLANDS

Thyroid: The thyroid gland lies near the Adam's apple and is the chief iodine storehouse of the body. It produces two important hormones: One is *thyroxine,* which speeds up the metabolism, and the other is *calcitonin,* which decreases the calcium levels in the blood.

The inner activity of your system is controlled by the thyroid gland. It is responsible for preventing the retention of water, sluggishness of the tissues, and densification of the bones. The proper development and function of the sex organs also depend on a normal and healthy thyroid. It is responsible for your poise, tranquility, and well-being. You can be either alert or dull, quick or slow, animated or depressed, all due to the activity of your thyroid.

Now let's talk about the thyroid reflexes. Using the thumb of the opposite hand, press along the inside edge at the base of the thumb. Work all around this area until you hit the reflex to the thyroid. If you have any kind of thyroid congestion, you will experience a sharp pain when you press it. The whole area may be quite tender, with the pain quite pronounced at first. Nevertheless, as you continue to work with a rolling-pressing motion, built-up crystals around the reflex will be broken loose and washed away by the increased flow of blood. You will notice the pain becoming less and less each time you do reflex work on this area. The thyroid is a very important hormone-producing gland and is not to be neglected, even if you do not feel the tenderness in this reflex that you might feel in other glands. Work it anyway.

Remember, do not get carried away and work any of these reflexes for a long period of time the first few days. You may find that the tenderness is not so sharp and painful in the hands as it is in the feet, due to the daily use of the hands.

For those who do not have my book *Healing Yourself with Foot Reflexology,* the thyroid reflexes on the feet can be found just at the base of the big toe, the same as at the base of the thumb. Be sure to work this reflex in both hands. If you work the foot reflexes, do both feet. Never leave half of the body untreated.

Parathyroids: There are four of these tiny glands, two embedded on each side of the thyroid gland. The glands influence the maintenance of the body's metabolic equilibrium. These small glands secrete the *parathyroid hormone,* which controls the body's supply of calcium and the content of phosphorus in the bones and the blood. People whose parathyroids are not working properly may develop twitching muscles and convulsions.

If you study the Endocrine Gland Chart on page 57, you will notice the location of the tiny parathyroid glands. In reaching the reflexes to these tiny glands, you will use the same position as you use to work reflexes to the thyroid, except you will have to reach a little deeper. The parathyroids will generally get enough stimulation when you work the reflexes to the thyroid, unless there is a definite congestion within them. If these glands need special attention, a reflex tool can be used for deeper pressure on the reflexes. The eraser end of a pencil or one of the hand reflex tools may be used. However, be careful how hard you press, as you do not want to bruise the tissues or capillaries in your hands. Work the reflexes in both hands.

Thymus: The thymus gland is located roughly level with the top of the breastbone. It is one of the lymph glands that helps dispatch white blood cells and fights infection. It is somewhat of a mystery gland, as it is very active during childhood, but by the time we reach adolescence, the thymus gland diminishes in size.

Scientists have found that the thymus helps make cells called *T-lymphocytes,* which have an influence on our immunity to disease and help fight off infections. The more the thymus is in malfunction, the more the body is subject to illness, especially in the young.

To reach the reflexes to the thymus, you should work the area next to the thyroid reflex at the base of each thumb. Also, work the inside of the index finger, on the beginning of the lung and bronchial reflex. The reflex to the thymus is located in an area where it will benefit from other reflex work. There is no reason to be concerned about the thymus, as long as the other endocrine glands are in harmony with each other.

Pancreas: The pancreas is another ductless gland that is responsible for keeping your body sugar at its proper level. It produces two hormones: *insulin* and *glucagon,* which separately decrease and increase the level of blood glucose, keeping it within set limitations. The pancreas also has an exocrine pancreatic duct that generates digestive enzymes.

The reflex to the pancreas is on the palm side of each hand, just below the reflex to the stomach. There are several very active organs within the abdominal area. Therefore, you will be working other reflex areas as you work the pancreas area.

For the person who has high or low blood sugar levels, this reflex area will be very sore. Stimulating the reflex to the pancreas can cause the blood sugar level to change very fast, so work with caution if you have diabetes or hypoglycemia. Check with your doctor if needed.

Adrenals: We have two adrenal glands, one on top of each kidney. They produce *corticosteroids* and *epinephrine.* These hormones regulate blood, influence our metabolism, and secrete sex hormones. They also produce *adrenaline,* which prepares us for crisis by increasing our heart and breathing rate, sending more blood to our muscles for instant energy if needed in the case of an emergency.

Your adrenal glands promote the wisdom of perception, the untiring activity, and the drive to action, the inner energy, courage, vigor, and the fervor expressed in every way. They intensify the flow of blood, its oxygenation, and organization powers.

Now you know how important healthy adrenal glands are to your well-being and happiness. To work the reflexes to each of these important glands, place your thumb on the reflex just above the kidney reflex on the palm side of each hand.

Gonads: These are the body's sex glands. The ovaries in women release *progesterone* and *estrogen* hormones, which control facial hair, breast size, and pregnancy. The testes in men release *testosterone*, the hormone that controls the production of sperm.

Truly, the gonads are the most important to your happiness of all the other ductless glands. The hormones secreted by these sex glands create the inner warmth in your system, preventing all tendencies toward inflexibility. They are responsible for your ability to attract people and keep their affection, and for making your personality radiant and magnetic. Sparkling eyes, self-reliance, and self-assurance are an indication that the gonads are functioning properly.

You can see on the Endocrine Chart the location of the gonads (ovaries/testes). Although they are located differently in the female and male body, you will use the same reflex area. Notice that the reflexes to these glands are located on the wrist of both hands, on the same side as the little finger.

Remember that the gonad glands are interrelated to all the other endocrine glands as well as the nervous system. The nervous system enables us to react quickly, whereas many of the hormones released by these significant glands are more durable and have longer-lasting effects on the body.

The word *hormone* comes from a Greek word meaning "excite." We know the rhythm of our body is controlled by hormones. The health of our endocrine glands can cause us to speed up or slow down; they can motivate us with excitement, or cause our mood to be depressed.

So work the reflexes in your hands (or feet) to keep these powerful coordinators of your body functions healthy and in complete balance. Use your fingers to search out sore spots and, when you find them, work them out, so you can live a healthy, happy, and harmonious life.

THE ENDOCRINE SYSTEM AND ITS REFLEXES

Chart G: All body functions take place because of the intricate interaction of various nerves and coordinating endocrine chemicals. Here you see the location of important endocrine glands in the body and their corresponding reflex areas in the hands. We will refer to these glands often as you study reflexology, so learn them well.

Reflexology Transforms Vital Life Forces into Activity

As I have stated before, your glandular system is the transmitter of vital life forces that are transformed into activity through the body. This is why any improper functioning of the endocrine glands can be normalized with reflexology.

Insufficiencies and imbalances of the endocrine glands are usually of a functional, not an organic, nature. This means that the glands are intact, but they suffer from an inadequate supply of nerve energy and nourishment, derived from an improperly oxygenated bloodstream.

Therefore, the purpose of working the reflexes to this system is to enhance the life forces and increase circulation in glandular areas, thus promoting renewed health and efficiency.

Reflexology Helps Dissolve Enlarged Thyroid

Dear Mildred,

I feel as though I know you as an old friend, even though we have never met. I am 74 years old but nobody thinks I look nearly that old. I would like to tell you what convinced me that reflexology really works. For many years, I had an enlarged thyroid, which was very visible. By using directions from your book on "Hand Reflexology" I actually rid myself of every trace. I have really been blessed with good health! Thank you and God Bless.

Yours to Good Health,

J. A. A.

Reflexology Helpful for Delinquent Children

Endra Devi tells us in her book *Forever Young, Forever Healthy* of an experiment made by Dr. Rowe in the course of which he found that moroseness, bullying, disobedience, lying, thieving, and vagrancy in children were often due to a faulty pituitary function. In the face of this information, if the technique of reflexology were used in the home by the entire family, we could have less child delinquency. She goes on to tell us that an increase of blood supply and nerve energy naturally improves and heightens the functional activities of the glands. I know this is true of

Yoga, and it is also true that we can accomplish the same results by working the reflexes to these very important endocrine glands.

Reflexology Keeps Glands in Tune

Remember that reflexology deals with the functions of life and the endocrine glands are the orchestra of your life. Keep them in tune by using reflexology, and your whole being will be in harmony with the symphony of the universe.

Strengthen Endocrine Glands for Natural Healing

Working reflexes that correspond to the endocrine glands help motivate natural healing energies. Nature has designed our body with these valuable glands to control our functions and rhythms by secreting a variety of chemical hormones directly into the bloodstream to boost our mobility, stabilization, energy, and organization of life processes. We hear spectacular recoveries from many who have used reflexology to help themselves, as well as relieve others, from pain and suffering and return to glorious health.

How a Victim of Muscular Dystrophy Was Helped in Minutes

When we were on a trip up the Northwest Channel of Canada, on a ferry, I noticed a quite attractive lady dragging her foot as she walked, her husband having to help her most of the time even though I could tell it hurt her to be so dependent on him. Some time later my husband joined her husband in a game of cards, so I went over and sat beside her. It wasn't long until she was telling me of her troubles.

Mrs. M. said that she had muscular dystrophy and the doctors told her there wasn't anything that could be done for her, and she would just have to be reconciled to becoming an invalid as the disease would progress slowly over her whole body. She was understandably depressed and very unhappy.

I asked her if she had ever heard of reflexology and she said that she hadn't. I told her a little about how it worked and asked her to let me massage her hand, which I did for about ten minutes and she was amazed at the results. She couldn't wait to tell her husband about it and how good it made her feel all over. I offered to give her a complete treatment later if she wanted me to do so. We made an appointment to meet them in their state-room where I massaged her hands and feet for about 20 minutes. We made a date to have dinner with them later.

When they came into the dining room, she was walking alone without a sign of a limp and her face was radiant. When the woman who was sharing their stateroom with them came in, she looked at Mrs. M. and asked what had happened to her. She was amazed at what they told her about reflexology.

Mrs. M. said that she was starved for the first time in months. Mr. M. and she could not believe the results that they were seeing happening before their very eyes in such a short period of time. And once again I thanked God for leading me to this wonderful method of bringing health to my fellow man.

This natural method of healing is safe and free for all to use. I hope you will put it to work to help not only yourself, but also to help others who are sent to you for relief from suffering and need the freedom from illness and pain.

How Reflexology Helped Multiple Sclerosis Victim

I started using reflexology treatments on my husband and myself, then it really grew out of hand. All of my acquaintances wanted me to massage their feet.

God led me to a 39-year-old woman suffering from multiple sclerosis. This method hasn't performed a miracle because only God can, but she is comfortable. Before treatments, she had to have shots in her knees. Her menstrual periods had stopped. Her skin was very scaly. Her bowels weren't performing. Happy to say, all these are cleared up. I have only been treating her a year, twice a week. She had been bed-ridden for 13 years before I met her.

I am sorry, but I have become disillusioned with the Medical Profession as a whole—very few old, good M.D.'s are left.

Mrs. D.A.

Parkinson's Disease Helped with Reflexology

Here is a miraculous story describing how one very dedicated man helped his mother-in-law keep Parkinson's disease under control.

He has shared his treatment techniques, which are very valuable. He also gets his message across, that reflexology comforts and contributes to healing. Mr. Chee shows us that we can overcome any challenge to our health with faith and patience. Let us celebrate his victory and give thanks for his accomplishments.

How Reflexology Helped Parkinson's Patient Recover

Dear Mrs. Carter,

I want to tell you of an extraordinary case of Parkinson's disease, which involved my mother-in-law, Chong Lee Yoke (age 75 at the time). Parkinson's affects the forebrain cells and causes an involuntary muscle movement. It leads to the characteristic tremor of the hands, with rigidity of the muscles and very slow movement. My mother-in-law suffered from this dreadful disease. When the forebrain collapsed, the whole body also collapsed, causing some sort of paralysis. One can never understand why she got it when all her glands were in tiptop shape.

It was rather bad for the first two weeks. At times, she used to talk nonsense. There was no time to stand and stare. Madame Chong was in semi coma state with Parkinson's disease, her brain cells in total collapse. She even could not recognize her sons and daughters. Luckily, reflexology came to the rescue. I quickly worked on the "watchdogs" of the body, the "endocrine glands," most of which were tender, especially the pituitary, thyroid, and adrenal glands. Time was then spent on the pineal, thymus, pancreas, and the gonads. Then I also tuned up the liver, kidneys, lungs, heart, spleen, and the solar-plexus network of nerves. A bit of time was also spent on the lymph glands.

When I tried to rejuvenate her feet and ankles, to release tension, they were very stiff. Then I proceeded to the spinal reflexes and the magical button "solar plexus," working forty minutes on both feet and ten minutes on the hand reflexes. She could not eat for the first three days. Then I added in more time on the webbing between the big toe and the second toe, with a good workout to the throat reflex.

I kept reflexing her every day, and she began to eat and feel conscious of her surroundings. She could recognize her sons and some visitors; she was on the road to recovery. Reflexology works miracles.

Within two months, she could walk with the aid of a walking frame. There were occasions, when her hand started to tremble, I went straight to the adrenal and pituitary reflexes, and when I gave the solar plexus an additional push, the hand ceased to tremble. This is something worth noting. Her rapid recovery was fantastic—reflexology did the trick again.

And in three months she baffled me. She could walk independently. But great credit must be given to her, as she is very determined, and every morning without fail, she walked three or four rounds in the garden. She did some hand swinging and breathing exercises like the Chinese art of "Tai Chi." There is no permanent cure for Parkinson's, and sometimes the hand starts to tremble again, but reflexology puts it back in order.

Today she is already 83, looking as strong as ever. Everything is shipshape. She can walk, eat, and do everything, thanks to the help of reflexology! My wife, mother-in-law, and I send our love to you and your daughter.

Yours lovingly,

Bobby Chee, Island Glades

CHAPTER 7

Treating the Eyes at Home with Reflexology

If nerves are fatigued, the muscles of the eyes function imperfectly, as eyestrain and tired muscles are largely under the control of the nervous system. Almost instant relief may be obtained by pressing reflexes on the second and third fingers, and holding the pressure for several minutes.

In treating eye weakness, there are several things to keep in mind, but give special attention to reflexes that might be involved in any of the following: blocked circulation to the eyes caused by tight muscles in the neck; a vertebra out of alignment; faulty kidneys; diabetes; or possibly other malfunctioning glands. So, when trying to overcome any type of eye trouble, be sure to check the eye reflexes and give particular care to those reflex areas mentioned above. Consult an eye specialist if your eye problems continue after a few weeks.

HOW TO LOCATE REFLEXES FOR THE EYES

For eye weaknesses, as noted on Chart B (page 11), the locations of the eye reflexes are just at the base of fingers two and three, where they meet the palm of your hand. Chart E (page 14) shows how the zone lines run from fingers two and three through the eyes. You can also help strengthen the eyes by using a firm pressure on the ends of these two fingers. Remember, if just one eye is involved, you will focus most of your reflex work in the hand and fingers on the side where the weak eye is located.

It will be helpful to use the reflex clamps to hold a steady pressure on the ends of these fingers to help manifest a vital life pulsation into the eye region, thus helping nature clear out any congestion that may be causing malfunction of some part in the delicate eye canals.

The reflexes in the thumbs may also be involved, so search for tender spots in them as well. Also, do some reflex work in the webbing between fingers.

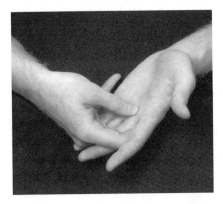

Photo 13: Apply a rotating pressure with your thumb at the base of the index and middle fingers on the left hand to stimulate healing circulation to the left eye.

Reflexes to Improve Eyesight

One of the most important things we can do for ourselves is to save our eyesight. Reflexology, exercise, good nutrition, and vitamin supplements all play an important part in preserving our vision so that we can enjoy a clearer view of the beautiful world we live in.

With the thumb of your opposite hand, press-and-roll along the base of each finger. Then work up and down each finger with the press-and-squeeze technique (see page 71) to energize all the zones. If you have sore or weak hands, you may want to use a self-help tool of some sort to stimulate the eye reflex points. You can use the eraser of a pencil or the Magic Reflexer to activate renewed circulation to the eyes. Start out by working the pressure buttons for only a few seconds, then come back and work each finger for one or two minutes at a time. Work them daily.

Also work the liver reflex area on your right palm and then work the reflex area of the adrenal and kidney on each hand to clear away any energy blockages within these zones. When the liver and kidneys are in poor health, eye problems can occur.

HOW TO RELIEVE EYESTRAIN

You will find that pressure on the lower and upper side (see Photo 5, page 32) of fingers two and three will relieve eyestrain in a few minutes. If there are certain nerves pinched in the neck, which lead to the eyes, reflexes in the thumbs should also be involved. Work the thumbs if you suffer frequent headaches from eyestrain. In addition, work the webbing between fingers, which corresponds to the sensory organs, and includes the eyes.

Use body reflexology to ease eyestrain: You will find some very sensitive reflexes around the eyes themselves, which you should also work on if you are having eye problems. These reflexes will be easy to find by their tenderness when you press on the right buttons.

On the outer edge of your eye, which will be in zone three or four, you will feel where the bone circles the eye. Now with your index or middle finger, gently press on the curve of this bone and feel for a sore reflex spot in this area, which will probably be right at the corner of your eye.

Now, using the same method, press on the bony area as it curves over the top of the eye. Search out the sore spots just as you would for a tender button in the fingers and hands.

Do the same under the eye, being sure to press on the *bony structure only.* You will find another tender reflex button to press, on the inner corner of the eyes, next to the nose. In fact, you may find several tender spots in this area along the nose. There is no need for heavy pressure in these areas, so *be very gentle.*

Remember, you are not to press into the eye, but on the bony structure surrounding it, using a careful, steady pressure or a very light rotating motion, whichever seems to be better for your particular need. End this reflex work by pressing along the temples, as well as across, and between your brows to reduce eyestrain.

Caution: Do not work on the eye reflexes for more than a few seconds, and never more than once a day for the first week or two, as these reflexes are quite powerful and might result in a headache.

Continue your reflex work and it will eventually eliminate your eye troubles. Keep in mind that your body has been years running down, so do not expect to build it up in a day.

Exercises to Renew Eye Health

The following two exercises can be done with your hands for renewing health of your eyes: Start by stretching your fingers. Open one hand, spread all fingers out as far as possible. Now starting with your little finger, fold it in toward the palm, let the other fingers follow to make a tight fist. Repeat several times on each hand.

The second exercise is to fold your hands together, interlocking each finger. Turn the fingers of one hand to the left, and fingers of the other hand to the right, applying pressure at the base of all fingers. Turn your fingers in the opposite direction and squeeze again. (See Illustration 13.)

These are excellent exercises to help improve eyesight because they stir circulation at the base of fingers, which is the exact spot of your eye and ear reflexes.

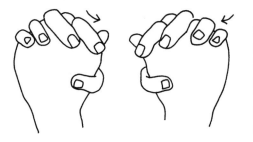

Illustration 13: Clasp hands together. Turn fingers to the left and squeeze, then turn fingers to the right and squeeze. This is an easy exercise to invigorate circulation to the sensory organs.

Reflexology is not costly or complicated: It is free and simple to use. Just fold your hands together and apply pressure at the base of all fingers. What could be easier? You can do this exercise anytime, anywhere, to help relax nerves and stimulate eye reflexes. Do it today and everyday, so you will be able to enjoy better vision tomorrow and forever.

HOW TO USE REFLEXOLOGY TO STOP EYE TROUBLES

Use the same pressure on the first, second, and third fingers to help clear up sties, burning of the eyes, and inflammatory conditions. These cases are completely relieved when pressure is exerted on reflexes in the fingers. Sties are frequently relieved in one or two treatments while other conditions may take longer.

Stop watery eyes: To reach the tear duct of the eyes, press on webbing between the second and third fingers. Push upward on the lower knuckle joint of the index finger to help stop watering eyes. Hold until weeping stops.

Cataracts helped with reflexology: I have had success in treating cataracts with reflexology on the feet alone. By using foot reflexology and the earlier mentioned hand methods, you, too, will get wonderful results and help bring health and sparkle back into your precious eyes.

Reflexology Helps Arrest Cataract

Dear Mrs. Carter,

About six months ago, my niece was told she had precataract condition of the right eye and thinning of the walls of both eyes. On recent checkups, there was a marked improvement and she was told not to come back for a year.

She told the doctor she had been using reflexology, and he agreed it was a good idea to continue it.

Thought you might be interested. I have been using it for two years and can't say enough praise for it.

Mrs. A.

Glaucoma Helped with Shiatsu and Reflexology

Dear Mrs. Carter,

I feel this will be of great interest to you. My auntie is suffering from glaucoma. I applied the reflexology around her eyes as in your Body Reflexology book, coupled with the Japanese massage "Shiatsu" and received unbelievable results that work like magic. After two treatments she could see and all her tensions on the eye vanished like a dream. She was so happy. In fact, a very famous eye specialist here advised her to have an operation, as glaucoma can cause blindness. Then my auntie asked me whether reflexology could help. I told her why not try it. All in all, I spent about one and one-half hours on each of her sessions. It is a great relief. Wishing you the very best of health and everlasting happiness.

With Love,

B. C.

How Eyestrain Was Relieved by Reflexology

Dear Mrs. Carter,

I want you to know that my health has greatly improved and I feel like a new person since practicing the suggestions outlined in your book *Healing Yourself with Foot Reflexology.*
Over the years the doctors have treated me for an enlarged heart, an overactive thyroid, impaired hearing, some arthritis in the fingers, and hemorrhoids. Three years ago I started with chiropractic treatments and found great relief. Now I am convinced that by following the methods outlined in your marvelous book, that all my discomforts will be eliminated.
Just a few days after receiving your book, I awoke one morning to find that I was unable to read the newspaper or other fine print. This was due to using my eyes for long periods of time on needlepoint work and much reading. After working reflexes in both feet for several weeks, my vision returned to normal.

Thank you for compiling this priceless book.

Mrs. A.T.

CHAPTER 8

How to Use Reflexology to Regain Hearing

It is hard to convince people that by pressing several reflex points in the fingers (or toes) that it will benefit hearing from the adjacent ear. Yet, this is a fact.

Physicians, familiar with the practice and principles of Zone Therapy (Reflexology), have used this method and claimed that nine out of ten cases of otosclerosis can be improved up to ninety percent. Otosclerosis is thickening of the ear membranes that immobilize one of the tiny bones in the ear, preventing the vibrations of sound. Reflexology helps correct ringing or hissing in the ears, and if there is any hearing left, you will almost certainly be able to improve it.

A very famous German music composer, Ludwig van Beethoven, was deaf from otosclerosis when he was about thirty years old. Beethoven lived in the early 1800s. However, if he was living in today's world, we would certainly try to help him hear again with reflexology.

REFLEX TECHNIQUES TO IMPROVE HEARING

A neighbor's son was in a rock band when he was in high school. The boys would close themselves in the garage and play their electric guitars and drums for hours at a time. By the time Don was 22, he noticed he had a hearing problem. Fortunately for Don, his mother gave him reflexology treatments, and evidence suggests his hearing condition has been corrected.

Many people who have hearing difficulties are greatly helped with the use of reflex therapy. Now you too can use this method to renew your own hearing health, by working the fingers on each of your hands.

Highlighting Reflex Zones to the Ears

Remember, the human body is not flat like the charts. When we talk about a zone, keep in mind that it takes in a large section from the front to the back of the body. Here we will concentrate on the zones affecting the ears. Let us start with the outer ear and follow the path of sound waves through the canals until they reach the brain. Refer to the Zone Chart on page 14.

Zone 5 travels from the end of each little finger, and corresponds to each outer ear where sound waves enter.

Zone 4 follows through the end of the fourth fingers, which represent a pathway of vital energy that flows to the ear.

Zone 3 runs from the third fingers. This zone is the channel that amplifies and carries sound waves through the ear canal and vibrates them off the eardrum.

Zone 2, found in the second fingers, designates the pathway to the inner ear that takes in and translates what you hear. Also within the inner ear is a fluid that vibrates tiny nerves, sending the sound messages to your brain.

Zone 1 is in line with your thumbs and corresponds to your brain, which interprets the information you hear.

When helping yourself with hand reflexology for the ears, make sure to treat the fingers of your left hand if it is the left ear that is troubling you, and the right hand if it is the right ear. Treat both hands if neither of your ears is functioning as it should.

Start your reflex work by applying firm pressure to the top of each finger. This sends energy to the sinus cavities, which ultimately may affect the extent of hearing. You can also use the Reflex Comb to press the tips of all the fingers (see Photo 61, page 285),

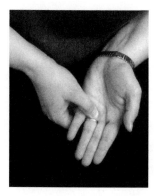

Photo 14: Working reflexes in the fourth finger zone on the left hand, stimulates a life force of healing energy to the left ear.

thus sending the healing life force into malfunctioning ears. Hold this pressure for about five minutes. Give deep pressure to the pituitary reflex point, which is located in the center pad of each thumb, to encourage stimulation to the brain.

Next we will work the webbing between all fingers, as these are the reflex areas of your sensory organs, which make you aware of things around you through sight, smell, touch, taste, and hearing. (See finger exercise on page 66 to help sensory organs.)

Also, work up and down each finger with a press-and-squeeze movement to clear pathways of the auditory nerves. Work each finger for several minutes at a time, repeating the procedure numerous times throughout the day.

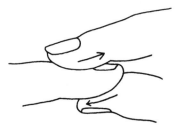

Illustration 14: Use a press-and-squeeze motion by pushing thumb forward, and at same time, pulling index finger backward. Work the full length of each finger with this technique.

Circulatory disorders within the ears often are the cause of hearing disturbances, balance problems, and dizziness. So, work completely around the base of each finger where it connects to the palm of your hand (see Photo 14), thus sending the healing life force into malfunctioning ears. Use reflex stimulation several times a day until all symptoms of ear congestion, deafness, ringing in the head, and so forth have disappeared.

Give a complete reflex workout to help improve hearing, searching for tender reflex areas as you go, because if one part of the body is out of balance, it will affect other areas. This is especially true with the endocrine glands; if they are out of balance, it could affect the normal process of your auditory passageways. Work the reflexes to these glands on both hands to harmonize their important activities. (See Chart G, page 57.)

If the ear seems to be plugged up, open your mouth wide at the same time you are working on the fingers. This helps open the ear canals, as your ears and throat are interconnected. Therefore, it will be helpful to work the reflex area that corresponds to your throat, which is located around the base of each thumb.

Remember, in order to maintain hearing improvement, it is vital that you be persistent with the reflex treatments. In some cases, if workout sessions are discontinued for any appreciable length of time, the condition sometimes returns. So even if your hearing has returned, do not neglect to use these reflex pressures often on the important little push buttons to the ears.

Continue treatment to benefit ears and continue to have patience with your body's healing process. Remember, it may have taken a long time to get into this condition, so allow it time to heal. Your goal is to relax tension and tone up the body first; then harmony and renewed health will be restored *naturally.*

How to Use Body Reflex Methods to Improve Hearing

In addition to the finger pressure, you can reach up and work the reflexes around your ears to encourage stimulation. Work all around the ear and pull down the lobes. Place the tip of your third finger behind the ear lobe, where it fastens to the neck. Here you will feel an indentation. This is a special reflex point that will most likely be very tender when pressed, so with a gentle rotating movement, apply soft pressure and send a healing force of energy surging to the internal ear canals.

There is a wide spectrum of causes for hearing problems; among them are imbalance within the inner ears, allergies, inflammations, and sinus inflammations. Ear troubles can even be caused from low or high blood sugar, or from crying hysterically. Even tooth or jaw misalignments have been known to cause annoyance in the ears. This situation causes a "sound" that only the person suffering can hear, called *tinnitus.* One man described this unchanging noise in his ear as the sound of a hundred small firecrackers continually going off.

Another time a student told me that the ringing in her ears comes and goes. She finds when her elimination, or bowels, are not working as they should, the ringing in her head starts and she hears noises like someone is broadcasting to her.

How Doctors Used a Special Reflex Point in the Mouth

Many doctors have used a body reflex point located in the mouth to help their patients regain hearing and dissolve the internal sounds they hear. This reflex point corresponding to the ear is located behind the wisdom tooth and can be stimulated with a steady pressure. The doctors advised their clients to bite down hard on an object, such as a sterilized hard rubber eraser. They placed the eraser in the space between the last tooth and the angle of the jaw for about five minutes, repeating treatment several times a day.

Caution: If you choose to place an object in your mouth, make sure to sit or stand while doing so. Never lie down with anything in your mouth, as it could become a choking hazard. Do not use this technique on children, the sick, or the elderly.

Osteopaths, chiropractors, and naturopathic doctors, who have not hesitated to use this method of healing, have frequently had some startling results. One doctor told us of a dentist who helped more than twenty of his patients hear better by using this simple, yet beneficial treatment of reflex pressure.

CASE HISTORIES FROM THE FILES OF VARIOUS DOCTORS

It does sound too simple and easy to be true, doesn't it? But let me give you a few case histories from the files of various doctors who have used these methods with such great success. It may then be easier to put the teaching into practical use and benefit from this simple technique of reflex therapy to free yourself of all ear troubles by squeezing and pressing the fingers for a few minutes, several times a day.

Doctor's Wife Hears after Thirty Years

The wife of an ear specialist was brought to me for treatment for deafness. The doctor had tried unsuccessfully every accredited method and was constrained to see what zone therapy could do.

For thirty years this patient had heard nothing with the right ear, and very little with the left. I stimulated with a curved cotton tipped probe the area lying between the last tooth and the angle of the jaw. After two treatments, this patient could hear a small tuning fork one-half inch away from the right ear and one inch from the left. After a few treatments, her hearing so wonderfully improved that she could hear a whisper with the right ear. Imagine this, after being deaf for thirty years, and after having visited all the noted aurists in this country and abroad.

Singer Recovers Hearing

A young soprano member of a leading Hartford church choir suffered a progressive loss of hearing, which finally became so pronounced as to make it almost impossible for her to "sing on the pitch," or harmonize with either the organ or the other quartet members.

She received treatment similar to that employed on the doctor's wife, supplementing it by "home treatment." This consisted of tucking a wad of surgeon's cotton or a solid rubber eraser in the space in back of the wisdom tooth, and having her bite forcibly upon it, repeating the procedure several times daily, especially immediately before singing or rehearsing. In a few weeks, this woman had completely recovered her hearing and was able to accept an engagement with a traveling concert company.

The doctor reporting on her case goes on to say, "I have had to date possibly fifty cases of deafness of one kind or another, all of whom have been helped materially."

Minister Cured from Otosclerosis in Minutes

One patient, a minister afflicted with otosclerosis for 25 years (supposed thickening of the membranes of the inner ear), could barely hear loud talking. After working for five minutes upon the joints of the third and fourth fingers, and to a lesser degree, upon the other fingers, it was found that the patient could hear a whisper twenty feet away.

As proof of this, it was whispered to him, "Will you close the window above your head?" He arose immediately from his chair and obliged.

How Physician's Relative Regained Hearing

A New York physician had a relative who had been unsuccessfully treated for deafness in one ear (the right) by conventional methods for the past 16 years, by some of the most famous aurists in New York, London, Paris, Berlin, Dresden, Vienna, and other centers of medical learning. X-ray treatment had at one time made this case at least 25 percent worse. With the left ear, this patient could hear a loud voice "close up."

Dr. Reid Kellogg volunteered to "show the doctor something," using this case for demonstration purposes. The doctor, like Barkis, being "willing," our friend took his trusty aluminum comb from his pocket and exerted pressure for five minutes with the teeth of the comb on tips of the patient's left hand. He also used the pressure in the mouth for an additional five minutes with a rubber eraser placed behind the wisdom tooth.

The doctor then stood ten feet away from his relative and talked to him in an ordinary tone of voice. The patient heard distinctly with the left ear every word spoken.

Our doctor then started to work on the other hand while the patient was protesting that this was a waste of time because some of the "biggest" ear specialists in Europe had failed to help the right ear. However, the attempt was made, and within ten minutes the patient heard a clock a foot away, a watch held three inches distant from his ear, and he further was able to repeat words spoken loudly two feet away. During the experiments with his right ear, the left ear was tightly plugged, so this test was quite conclusive.

Deaf Parents Made to Hear with Reflexology

A lady and her husband who were both deaf came to this doctor, but the baby in her arms was not deaf, and most decidedly was smart. Within two weeks' treatment, both parents could hear the baby cry every night, which was a great satisfaction to them in one way—but they don't know yet whether to laugh or cry about it!

Have you read enough to convince you of the wonderful results of reflexology for the ears? Let me quote two more case histories.

Hearing Returned to Deaf Soldier

A veteran who had been deafened by a gun concussion was treated by using the pressure behind the teeth on the gum margins near the angle of the jaw. He was then able to hear for the first time in years. That it was a pleasure was evidenced by the fact that the old soldier danced around the office in a perfect transport of glee.

Skeptic Cured after 39 Years of Deafness

One lady, aged 45, deaf since she was six years old, came to the office of a specialist who studied Zone Therapy (Reflexology). When the physician applied a comb to one hand, she whispered "crank" to a friend. Twenty minutes later, being able to hear ordinary conversation, she whispered "wizard."

HOW TO EASE AN ACHING EAR

We have found one of the most effective and quickest cures for an earache to be pressure exerted on the end of the fourth finger (ring finger) for about five minutes.

To start the vital life forces activating the congestion that has been causing the trouble, hold a steady pressure on the tip of the ring finger of the hand that is located on the same side as the aching ear. Keep this pressure on the finger until the ear stops aching or you can get to a doctor.

HELP FOR GRADUAL HEARING LOSS

Deafness is seldom sudden but creeps in so subtly that we refuse to acknowledge the condition as if it were some kind of disgrace. To keep a continuous watch over its possible onset, test your hearing by listening to your watch tick. If you can't hear it, chances may be that you are already "hard of hearing."

How a Socialite Regained Hearing

Mrs. L.P., a rich proud socialite, was unable to tell if her expensive watch needed repairs since she could not hear its usual ticking. Only then did she realize that her hearing was at fault, even though she blamed her inability to catch other sounds to distracting noises, and occasional failure to distinguish words, to poor speech. The discovery was a great shock and source of unhappiness, since she did not want to be forced to wear a hearing aid or be suspected of oncoming senility. One of her friends, who had cured her own partial deafness, told her about her experience with reflexology.

Mrs. L.P. took her friend's advice and immediately started using reflexology as directed by her friend. Her hearing was soon restored to normal, thus preserving not only her health but also her vanity.

Being "hard of hearing" or totally deaf is a serious affliction, not only for the sufferer, but a source of callous impatience and lack of compassion on the part of others, if not outright derision. The old-fashioned ear trumpet is still a prime source of comedy. It is no wonder that we hesitate to acknowledge its onset. Even with our advanced and modern designs of hearing aids, there are many who refuse to wear them.

Now, however, thanks to the miraculous healing power of hand, foot, and body reflexology, we can treat hearing loss promptly without expensive hearing aids, medication, or special equipment.

You Can Help Hearing Loss in Children

Hearing loss in children is often overlooked, even in these modern days of testing in schools. It has been learned that poor hearing may be the cause of poor speech since the child is unable to hear spoken words clearly, or of low grades because he is unable to hear the teacher. The child needs understanding and help, not scolding or accusations. To guard your child's emotional and physical health, a simple reflexology treatment once a week may help to insure perfect hearing in the future and a happy well-adjusted life.

You can teach him to use reflexology on himself, as most children enjoy using this natural way to help themselves maintain good health.

CHAPTER 9

How to Work Reflexes in the Tongue

In reflexology, there are various points that activate the body's healing forces. There are reflex buttons in the hands, feet, ears, body, and even in the tongue. Yes, there are a few reflex buttons in the mouth, which seem to abate distress and enhance stimulation to some areas of the body in certain situations.

Dr. Fitzgerald claimed the tongue had reflexes in it that follow along the meridian lines, just as in the body. Thus, zone one would be down the center of the tongue, with zone two extending out on each side. (See the Zone Chart on page 14.)

This is why some doctors tell us if there is a crack down the middle of the tongue, it indicates tension in the spinal area. Moreover, small cracks in the tongue can mean dry areas in the colon. The color of the tongue has a medicinal meaning also. A white surface symbolizes excess toxins and mucous in the body, and a yellowness signifies liver or gall bladder trouble.

However, your interest is in learning how to use the reflexes to help alleviate pain and illnesses in specific situations when needed. This technique of stimulating the reflexes in the tongue will be used in several instances throughout ensuing chapters. Therefore, you will want to know the method of activating these tiny reflex zones.

HOW ENTERTAINERS USE REFLEXOLOGY TO KEEP THEIR VOICES BEAUTIFUL

First, let us learn the art of pulling the tongue out as far as possible. Take a clean cloth between the fingers, stick the tongue out, and then take hold of it, using the cloth to hold it firmly. Now pull the tongue out as far as possible, and move it slowly from one side to the other for a few seconds.

Many of our great entertainers, including singers, use this method of stretching and reflexing the tongue to help keep their voices beautiful. It eases throat tension and frees the voice.

It is helpful for stopping a sore throat and even a cold. In this way you are employing stimulation to the first, second, and third meridian lines. These regions govern the function of vocal cords, larynx, and the respiratory passages.

Stretching, or pressing, the tongue to stimulate zones one, two, and three is also helpful when there is illness caused by malfunctioning cells in corresponding areas of the body. Reflex pressure on the tongue is especially beneficial to those who can only eat soft foods due to bad teeth or illness. Tongue reflexes are naturally stimulated when we eat hard foods such as apples and most salad foods, carrots, radishes, cucumbers, cereals, nuts, and even crunchy cookies.

HOW TO FIND ZONES IN THE TONGUE

Next, we will learn how to press down on the tongue farther back in the mouth for added stimulation in specified cases. You may need to use a probe to reach the reflexes farther back on the tongue. If you find yourself gagging, start closer to the front end of your tongue and work back a little at a time.

If you have one of our special Tongue Cleaning Wands, you will not have any trouble reaching back as far as you need to on the tongue. The wand has an open-ended cleaning edge, so it does not cause a gagging reaction. Moreover, the handles convert into both a probe and a small reflexer made just for the tongue. (See Photos 64 and 65, on page 286.)

When pressing the center of your tongue, note that you are stimulating the reflexes in zone one, the same zone as when pressing the thumbs (or toes). Reflexes found within zone one of your tongue correspond to your throat, neck, and spinal column.

If you move the probe over a bit to the left or to the right, you will be in zone two. Move it over a little more, and you will be in zone three. You will be amazed at the tender spots you will find in your tongue as you use pressure in different places.

Using tongue pressure should be done in conjunction with hand reflexology. Work on the first, second, and third fingers of each hand. (Or work on the first, second, and third toes if you are doing foot reflexology.)

Combining body, hand, foot, ear, and tongue reflex work is refreshing to the whole system. It adds stimulation of the electrical life force in various areas of the body where the meridian zone lines pass through.

CHAPTER 10

How Reflexology Helps the Jaw and Teeth

Is there a more unbearable pain than a jaw or toothache? And it usually strikes in the middle of the night or on a weekend when no doctor or dentist is available. This is where reflexology comes to the rescue. When in pain from an aching tooth or jaw, you would do most anything to stop it. But *what* to do is the question.

HOW TO STOP AN ACHING TOOTH WITH REFLEXOLOGY

If you have a painful tooth, and it is in the front of the mouth on the left side, then you need to pick up your left hand. You can see by look-ing at the Zone Chart (page 14) that the lines from the thumb and the index finger on the left hand go through the front teeth. So you should start working on the left thumb and index finger to deaden the pain.

If the toothache is on the right side, in back of the mouth, then you should follow the lines running down the right side, from fingers three, four, or five, according to where the painful tooth is located. After locating the approximate area of pain, you will start to work the reflex in the fingers lying in the correct zone lines.

If the tooth is causing you severe pain, put pressure on these reflexes using a reflex comb, or even dig your fingernails in. I have known people to use their front teeth to hold pressure on the reflexes in the corresponding fingers until the pain subsided. Pres-sure of a rubber band has been used, too, but you must keep a close eye on the finger—if it starts to turn blue, remove the rubber

81

band immediately. If you have the reflex clamps, you can use them successfully.

When the pain has subsided, take time to search on the fingers, and even the toes, for definite sore spots. When you find them, this will indicate the exact reflex to work, or hold with pressure, until you can get to a dentist. You should find that this will anesthetize any area that is on the meridian line running from the head to the connecting finger or toe.

Pressure should be used from three to twenty minutes: In one case where the patient had suffered all night, ten minutes of pressure on both sides of his index finger was used, and within that time all pain stopped. Anesthesia will last from ten to twenty minutes.

Work the Reflex on the Same Side of the Body as the Pain

My friend Bobby told me that he was having a disagreement about reflexology; this is what he had to say:

> Sometimes people are judged more by performance than by experience; for instance, it's like the roadside mechanics. It is often that they do a better job than the big car companies' mechanics. And the same is true with reflexologists. There are several books besides yours on the market. But they are a far cry from your wonderful presentations. Sometimes the more books you read, the more confusing it becomes. Some books have the reflex areas all mixed up.
>
> One person told me if you have pain on the right side, you have to massage the left foot. How very strange. Quite recently, I argued with her on this point. I explained that reflexology works on the zone lines. Right side pain, right foot, and left side pain, left foot. She still insisted she was right. Then I told her your toothache theory with a rubber band to prove the point. Finally one day, her friend got a severe toothache and she applied the theory of yours on the same side of body. It worked. Now she is convinced. All at once, she speeded away to buy your three books. What do you know . . . she is now one of your admirers.

HOW TO STOP AN ACHING JAW WITH REFLEXOLOGY

If you suffer with temperomandibular joint syndrome (TMJ), you will follow the Zone Chart (page 14) from the side of pain to the corresponding reflex. TMJ usually is the result of muscles tensing up in the jaw area. Pain is often in the jaw, neck, ear, eye, and head. Some doctors tell us that rheumatoid arthritis can cause this syndrome; however, it will be obvious in other parts of the body, if this is the case. To relieve jaw pain, refer to toothache relief and to other chapters on earaches, headaches, and arthritis.

Using body reflexology directly over the jaw will help release tension. Use a pressing, circular motion with the fingertips, right over the jaw muscle that hurts. If the jaw hurts on both sides, place the heels of both hands on jaws and apply firm pressure. Do this as you inhale a few slow, deep breaths. Then work on each side separately.

Work the reflex points on the face located in front of the ear. You will feel an indentation here. Use index and/or middle finger and place pressure in the indentation, holding for one minute while you take in a few very deep breaths. Move your fingers along the upper jawbone, stopping every half inch or so, to repeat pressure on the reflex points. Using this technique, work all the way to your mouth, just under your nose, as well as around your nose. Now work the lower jaw in the same way. If your jaw hurts on both sides, repeat this procedure on the other side also.

Work the indentation behind the ear, at the end of your jawbone. Hold and rotate pressure on this point to relax the jaw muscles. Repeat two or three times a day.

Health tips to help stop TMJ pain: Make sure you are not sleeping with your neck in a crooked position, and be careful not to twist your head to one side when on the telephone, or when reading. Do not eat hard candy or other foods that cause stress on the jaws. If you suspect that you are grinding your teeth at night, ~~buy a sport mouth guard. You will need to take a pair of scissors and cut it down to fit comfortably into your mouth, then place it between your teeth at night.~~ This will stop the tooth grinding, and just might stop your TMJ pain. *Practice Yoga, meditation, sports, Deal with the issues that produces it.*

HOW TO KEEP BONES AND TEETH HEALTHY

I have stopped many cases of toothache by searching out tender spots on the toes and fingers, then working them until the pain stopped. I also highly recommend using the Tongue Cleaning Wand to help

if is bacterial need antibiotics, if virus.
GLUCOSAMINE with condroitn!

keep bacteria and food particles off the teeth. Cavities and gum disease often cause infections and toothaches. Did you know that the tongue traps food particles, which decompose and form plaque? The bacterial plaque settles on your teeth and solidifies into a hard substance called tartar, which eats away at the teeth. Moreover, tartar can only be removed completely by dental professionals. So, take care of your teeth by brushing, flossing, and cleaning your tongue.

Modern dentists tell us that it is possible for teeth to grow back to health if given a chance. Studies show that teeth and jawbones have become denser and much stronger after taking calcium supplements for six years. Other doctors, such as Lennart Krook, D.V.M., Ph.D., and Leo Lutwak, M.D., Ph.D., of Cornell University, tell of carrying out a study of 80 people ranging in age from 21 to 68, who were given calcium supplementation over a period of a year which resulted in significant increases in bone density in the jaw.

Another dentist tells of treating his patients with calcium and relieving them of all types of tooth diseases. The teeth actually healed themselves when nature was called in to do her work.

Now we can easily understand how reflexology helps renew circulation to help heal our teeth and jawbones. Together with the proper supplements and a little knowledge of their needs, you may be able to keep healthy bones and teeth for as long as you live.

How a Doctor Cures Sore Teeth with Reflexology

Dr. Roemer reports a case of a man suffering from teeth so sore that he could not close his mouth. "I found sore spots on the inside of the thumb and first finger and made pressure on them with a comb," he goes on to tell us. "In about five or six minutes, I had him talking about his business, I then asked him how his teeth were." He was surprised to find most of the pain gone. "What did you do?" he asked. I showed him how to apply the pressure on his fingers and also how to use the comb for lasting relief from any further pain. A more thankful and grateful patient I have rarely seen, thanks to Dr. Fitzgerald's discovery of Zone Therapy (Reflexology).

The Ca helps producing secundarie dentit protectic the nerve. But decayed tissue must be clean up and replaced with biological material like tooth.

CHAPTER 11

How to Work Reflex Areas for Lung and Respiratory Problems

Let us look at Charts A and B (pages 10 and 11) and see the position of the lungs; notice how they lie in the chest, then notice how the reflexes to the lungs are situated along the pad under the fingers. You will notice the lungs take up a large space in the chest area. Moreover, the reflexes to the lungs take up a large portion in the upper part of the palm.

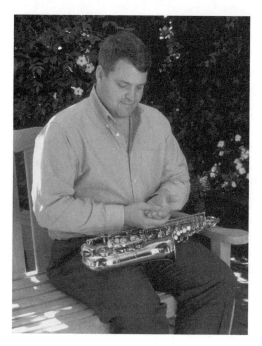

Photo 15: Position for stimulating the reflex area of the lungs. Work pads under the fingers on both hands.

The best position for working the lungs is to take your left hand and place it in the right hand. Using the right thumb, work along the reflexes on the pad under the fingers. Use a press-and-rotate or a walking-pressure motion as you work this whole reflex area. Work back and forth, and also up and down, so that the whole area will be stimulated.

You can also work diagonally in a criss-crossing movement to cover the lung and bronchial reflex area on each hand. Change hands and work in the opposite direction across your right hand.

The respiratory system is of major significance to good health, so let's use another method of reaching these important reflexes. With fingers on one side of the hand and the thumb on the other (see Photos 15, page 85 and 30, page 185), use a press-and-roll technique and work the reflexes on both sides of your hand simultaneously.

If you have one defective lung, then you will concentrate your reflex work on the hand that is on the same side of the body, working the tender reflex spots. However, just because one lung is affected, do not neglect to also work the other hand completely.

If your fingers are weak, you can use the eraser end on a pencil or a self-help reflex tool. Rolling your hands over the Deluxe Hand & Foot Roller would be beneficial.

THE IMPORTANCE OF THE RESPIRATORY SYSTEM

The respiratory system is more important to the perfect functioning of our whole body than most people realize. The trachea (windpipe), mouth, collarbone, bronchi, and lungs are all parts of this remarkable system. Together they deliver oxygen, from the air we breathe, into the bloodstream. The blood transports purified oxygen to the cells of which our bodies are built.

Working at the base of fingers and thumbs and between the webbing will benefit the upper respiratory system. Working the reflex of the lungs will also benefit the bronchial tubes.

The diaphragm muscle (and muscles from the ribs) moves the lungs as we breathe. When we breathe in, the diaphragm contracts and air rushes into the lungs. When we exhale, the diaphragm relaxes and moves up toward the lungs, forcing the air up and out of the windpipe.

Your lungs consist of millions of elastic membrane sacs, which together can hold about as much air as a basketball. Do you breathe in that much air, enough to keep your lungs full? The lungs are constantly inflating and emptying in their crucial capacity as a medium of exchange.

Your lungs sustain your life by unloading carbon dioxide and taking in oxygen carried by the blood to the cells. Oxygen unlocks the energy contained in your body's fuels. Do you know that your body's trillions of cells require so much oxygen that you need about thirty times as much surface for its intake as your entire skin area covers? Your lungs provide this surface area even though they weigh only about $2^{1}/2$ pounds. During moderate activity all the blood in your body passes through your lungs more than a hundred times an hour.

Can you see now why your lungs are one of the most important organs in your body? You could live several days without water, and several weeks without food, but you cannot live even several minutes without air. It is the "air of life" that nourishes the nuclei of all atoms, of all organs in the body.

This air, at all times present and perpetual, is the Creative Substance of all matter! This takes us back to Anaximenes (sixth century B.C.) who said: "The essence of the Universe is in the Infinite Air in eternal movement which contains ALL in itself."

When you were born you breathed in the breath of life immediately or you wouldn't be here today. Are you now beginning to understand the importance of a healthy respiratory system?

Faulty Lungs Cause Body Imbalance

Anyone who has any malfunctioning of the lungs naturally has some imbalance in other parts of the body as well. If one gland or organ is out of function, then it throws all the internal systems off balance, and we end up with a body that is out of harmony with the cosmic vibrations of the universe. Therefore, we can see that for any malfunction, no matter how small, we must treat the whole body, putting all the instruments back in tune to get a perfect melody.

This is the reason reflexology seems to be such a miraculous way to health. We do not treat just one malfunctioning part, we treat the whole unique individual for complete healing progress and renewed health.

Healing Exercises for the Lungs

Rejuvenating the lungs: Stand with your back straight and feet shoulder-width apart. With elbows straight, place your hands behind your lower back and clasp them together. Exhale air out of your lungs. Now inhale slowly and, as you do, open your hands and gently lift them up and away from your body. This will expand your lungs and open the chest, so that you can take in more air. As you continue to inhale, lift your hands and move them out in front of you. Raise them over your head if you can. Slowly return them behind your back as you exhale and repeat the exercise. Start doing this once a day and increase each day, until you are doing seven rounds in one rhythm.

You can add to this exercise of rejuvenating the lungs. Think positive thoughts as you inhale, and think of breathing out old stale used air as you exhale. This exercise is known to invigorate the whole breathing system.

Energizing the lungs: Sit down for this exercise as it can make you dizzy. After you inhale, push your shoulders back and think of your lower ribs widening as you hold the air for about five seconds, slowly release air and allow your diaphragm to push the air out of your lungs. Those who cannot get out of bed can do this exercise lying down. You can consciously open up your ribs by imagining that you are widening them as you breathe in. This exercise helps to oxygenate the entire system.

The panting exercise: Another way to get new fresh air into the lungs is to simply open your mouth, stick out your tongue, and breathe in-and-out very quickly. Renewed oxygen helps the body replace old cells with new and gives it added strength to heal itself.

HOW REFLEXOLOGY SPEEDS THE HEALING PROCESS

When we press on all of the reflex buttons, we are charging the whole body with a vibrating force of electric energy that promptly stimulates nature into a faster process of healing.

So you can see why you will always give yourself a complete reflex workout at least every other day while trying to stimulate one certain area that is in malfunction from congestion of one kind or another. This is where the magic of the little Magic Reflexer comes in. It can press and stimulate most of the reflex buttons in the hand at one time, not only to the lungs but to most of the organs and glands in the body.

If you are treating the lungs, you can use the Magic Reflexer once or twice a day on both hands. (Never take a half treatment.) Hold it in one hand while you squeeze and roll it around and around, pressing the little fingers into every reflex button in your hand. Now do the same with the other hand. You must not use it over two or three minutes at a time for the first two weeks.

HOW WE KNOW THE BENEFITS OF REFLEXOLOGY ARE REAL

When people are told of the wonderful results produced by reflexology, the first thing they say is, "Oh, it is just psychosomatic (all in the mind)." Doctors who do not understand the scientific art of reflexology use this as the only answer, but when you tell them it works as well on *animals,* they have to change their minds. Animals certainly don't know what you are trying to do when you use pressure on certain reflexes to anesthetize ailing parts of their bodies.

Your mind can influence your body: It cannot be denied, however, that the power of one's mind does influence the condition of the body, but an illness that is induced by wrong thinking is not *imaginary*—it is *real.*

We are constantly reminded of all kinds of terrible diseases by way of television, newspapers, magazines, and even advertisements on our computers. Consequently, we are being brainwashed to be illness prone.

How Your Thoughts Can Control Your Future

If the mind dwells on any illness for a certain period of time, the body is being conditioned for that disease and in a matter of time will accept what the mind has been preparing it for; and it then materializes. This is a scientific fact. We all know that our thoughts do control our future, for good or for bad, depending on how we direct them by conscious effort.

You can build a happy, healthy future: As I stated in my book *The Power of Thought,* "What you thought yesterday, you are living today; what you think today, you will live tomorrow."

Your thoughts have more power than you realize, and when you use them for health combined with the healing power of reflexology, you can live the rest of your life in the joy of perfect health.

Animals Show Proof that Reflexology Really Works

If you read my book on Foot Reflexology, you may remember the story about Inky, our little black Pomeranian who had asthma attacks. I gave his little paws several reflexology workouts. Sometimes he would jerk his foot away from me but would quickly put it back into position. He knew I was doing the one thing that would help him. It did not take long before he was completely healthy, and never had another attack of asthma.

Animals benefit from reflexology. They are proof that the results obtained are real, not mental. Animals do not know what is being done to them when we use reflexology to help them. Therefore, their minds could not have influenced the results that are obtained when reflex techniques are applied. Touching is a significant healing technique for pets as well as for people, and this includes reflexology's regenerating procedures.

How Reflexology Saved a Little Dog's Life

Dear Mrs. Carter,

I have had asthma and heart trouble for several years with a constant cough. Someone told us to get a Chihuahua dog and keep it near me at all times and it would help. So, three years ago my son gave me a present of a darling, tiny Chihuahua puppy. I kept him in my pocket when I was working and on my lap when sitting down, and to our surprise my symptoms vanished. Then "Wee Bits" started having spells of asthma. The veterinarian said there was nothing he could do for him. I just couldn't think of losing my little pet and it hurt me to see him suffer. All I could do was pray.

Then one day my daughter bought your book *Helping Yourself with Foot Reflexology,* and the first thing I turned to was your experience with your little dog that had asthma. God had answered my prayer! I started rubbing "Wee Bits's" feet just as you said you did to your dog. He seemed to enjoy the treatment and it was like a miracle. My little dog started to breathe normally in just a few minutes. Now all signs of his asthma attacks have stopped and he is once again healthy and full of energy. Your wonderful book saved my little dog's life.

I also use the treatment on myself and all of my friends. We are all thankful to you for writing this wonderful book showing us the positive, yet simple, way to help ourselves to stay healthy nature's way.

Mrs. S.

CHAPTER 12

How You Can Abort a Cold and Stop Coughs

Knowledge of the healing principles of reflexology is spreading throughout the world. The time is not too far distant when all people will be able to cure coughs and colds for themselves, without the dangers of medications.

If you have a bad cough, then try pressing on your thumb, as well as the first and second fingers, or the webbing between them. These reflexes may be stimulated by a steady pressure held on them for about ten minutes at a time. Reflex clamps can be used here with good advantage.

Remember that the throat is located in the first zone, which is the thumb; this is why we concentrate on the thumb and the fingers next to it for any problems of the throat. Next we would use the tongue probe to press and reflex the center of the tongue, which is also zone one, for five or ten minutes. I have cured many sore throats by just working at the base of the big toes and around the base of both thumbs.

How a Friend Was Cured of a Cold

I went to visit a dear friend and found her in bed suffering from a bad cold and a very sore throat. Her fever was high but she had refused to let anyone call a doctor.

I immediately went to work, first applying spring clothespins to the ends of all her fingers since I had nothing better with me.

I next fixed old-fashioned onion poultices and put them on her chest and her back. Then I uncovered her feet and went to work on all of the area around the big toe and the toes next to it.

I especially concentrated on the reflexes to the pituitary gland, located in the center of the big toe, and also in the center pad of the thumb. The other reflexes I left alone, as her body was trying to throw off enough poisons without stirring up more for it to take care of.

In less than an hour, Jessy was feeling much better and fell into a natural sleep, not waking until the next morning. Her fever had dropped to almost normal before I left for home. The next day, much against my advice, Jessy was up doing her work, feeling fine, except for being a little weak. She still says I was sent to save her life that day I made an unexpected visit.

The benefits of this reflex therapy are so powerful that it has cured many cases of the dreaded whooping cough in the days before vaccinations. Whooping cough is still not unheard of and it behooves everyone to learn the simple remedy of reflexology.

How Dr. Fitzgerald Cured Whooping Cough in Five Minutes

Whooping cough is one of the simplest and most easily-cured diseases with which zone therapy (reflexology) has to contend. An ordinary case of whooping cough, which has persisted for weeks, can sometimes be cured in from three to five minutes. Rarely are more than four or five treatments necessary. After the application of a probe held down firmly on the back of the tongue, little patients who had whooped themselves into a state of nervous and physical exhaustion never had another paroxysm of coughing.

Dr. Fitzgerald offered to demonstrate the method on one or one hundred cases and prove that, in one to a half dozen treatments, whooping cough can be effectively and permanently overcome.

The doctor stated, "In the several cases of whooping cough treated, we have not yet seen a failure from the proper application of zone therapy (reflexology)."

How a Woman Stopped a Stranger's Cough

Mrs. L. tells of going into town to do her shopping and noticed a woman standing by her car coughing: "She seemed to be coughing rather hard. I was concerned but didn't like to be bold so I went on into the store. When I came out about

15 minutes later, the woman was still standing in the same place coughing harder than ever. After putting my groceries in the car I went over to her and said, 'Would you like to have me tell you how to stop that cough?' She looked at me hopelessly and shook her head 'yes' as she continued the paroxysm of coughing.

"I told her to place her thumb on the lower joint of the first finger and to press hard. She looked at me kind of queerly but followed my directions. The cough seemed to subside almost immediately. I waited a few minutes to make sure it didn't start again, then I left. The last I saw of the woman she was still standing in the same spot holding her finger."

THE TRACHEA (WINDPIPE) AND HOW IT WORKS

Let us look at the rest of your respiratory system which consists of two large tubes, one for each lung, leading off the trachea (or windpipe), that taper on down into smaller bronchi tubes to make a tree-like formation within the lungs. You can see how disastrous it is for the body when a severe infection of these muscular bronchi results in destruction of the muscle necessary for contraction.

You will stimulate this part of your respiratory system as you work the reflexes for the lungs and voice. For special treatment of this area, you should concentrate on the thumb and first finger. Also, you can use tongue pressure.

DO NOT OVERWORK REFLEXES FOR COLDS

A cold is nature's way of cleaning house; I mean eliminating the system of acid. It is trying to rid the body of accumulated poisons, through mucous membranes in the head, nose, sinuses, and through pores of the skin. If your system is in perfect order, you will not be susceptible to colds or the various types of flu and viruses that spread through the country every few months. Do you ever wonder why some people catch everything that comes along and others seem to be happily immune and are never sick?

If you stay healthy all the time and never catch a cold, then your body is not burdened with poisons. However, if you do have colds frequently, then your body is overburdened, trying to eliminate toxic poisons. Therefore, you will not want to work all of the reflexes at this time, because it would only add further to its efforts in throwing off accumulated poison.

When you concentrate on working the reflexes that correspond to the head and lung area, you will be giving nature a little help, instead of hindrance, in clearing up your cold. You may give the kidney reflexes a very short workout to help them in their work of eliminating poisons the cold is trying to throw off. In the case of a fever, work the reflex to the pituitary gland in each thumb.

Helpful Tips to Avoid a Cold

There are many different cold viruses, each with its own symptoms and complications. The average cold lasts from two to seven days. The best way to avoid exposure to a cold virus is to take caution. Try not to touch your eyes, nose, or mouth when you are around others with a cold, and remember to wash your hands frequently, especially before you eat. Using your Tongue Cleaning Wand before and during a cold is essential for removing nasal drip, mucus, and harmful bacteria from the back of your tongue, and keeps your breath fresh.

Echinacea extract and supplements of Ester-C with bioflavonoids are two excellent immune stimulants. They also work as an antibiotic for colds, flu, hayfever, and infections.

In our family, when we have a cold or sore throat, we like to take one tablespoon each of lemon and honey in very warm water. We find it very soothing and it seems to help us rest, which the body needs for healing. We drink lots of fresh juice and other liquids to help fight germs and flush out toxins and infections. Warm broth, herbal tea, and chicken soup help break up mucus, and speed healing.

Sometimes putting Tea Tree Oil (or Eucalyptus Oil) on a cloth, or into a steamer, will make it easier to breathe. I find that the smell of Tiger Balm helps clear my nasal passage. And remember, to prevent spreading germs to others, always cover your sneeze, please.

How Reflexology Saved Child from Rheumatic Fever

Robert A. reports how he saved his daughter from the effects of rheumatic fever. "When my daughter, Sally, first became ill I didn't think too much about it," said Robert. "She had a sore throat for a few days; her mother was away taking care of her sister and new baby in another state. Sally, the boys, and I always got along fine for a few days without her. But when Sally started to run a high fever I became panic-stricken.

"I called the family doctor who is one of those rare physicians who still makes house calls. When he arrived, he took one look at Sally and said, 'Strep throat, which could cause rheumatic fever and damage her heart, if her fever runs too high.' He gave me some medication and warned me to watch her closely, and if the fever went higher to call him immediately. And he said I had better call her mother.

"I put in an emergency call to my wife and when I told her of our troubles she wasn't one bit upset. Mary was always a sensible girl and knew how to keep her cool, as the boys say. 'Sally is all right,' she told me calmly. 'You use reflexology on her and the fever will go down.'

"Reflexology had become a by-word in our house where sickness was concerned. Mary's mother had used it to keep her family healthy for many years, having learned it from a neighbor. I felt the tensions of fear lift and I asked her what she wanted me to do. 'Massage the reflexes to the pituitary to take the fever down,' she said. 'This is the little spot that is so sore in the center of your big toe a lot of times.' I knew the spot! 'Also work on the thumb and web of both hands. But keep at it, do it every few minutes until the fever goes down. The boys can help you. Don't massage anyplace else. I can't get home before late tomorrow, but Betty is okay now and can take care of the baby. Bye-bye!'

"The boys did help. We rubbed that little spot in the center of Sally's toes and thumbs every few minutes all night long. It was breaking dawn when the fever went down to near normal.

"The next morning when the doctor came by to check on Sally, he was amazed at her quick recovery. 'She really had me worried,' he said. We told him what my wife had told us to do. He shook his head sadly and said, 'Too bad more people don't know how to use reflexology, it would save me a lot of work, and many families a lot of heartache.'"

How a Bronchial Cough Was Stopped

A patient with a bronchial cough, under my instruction, relieved her cough by pressures made on her tongue, around the base of her thumbs, and index fingers.

This lady reported the following morning that she had enjoyed her first night's sleep in more than five nights, and that a persistent and annoying headache had also cleared up.

These results are quite uniform and can be duplicated by anyone. Indeed this procedure is so simple that I have repeatedly seen bronchial and other coughs resulting from irritation or congestion at some point in the air passages, completely cured, merely by pressure on the tongue, which had persisted for a long time.

Don't underestimate the wonders of reflexology in any field of healing! If medical doctors have used and praised it so highly, then you can be thankful that the knowledge of this tremendous field of natural healing has been revealed to you.

CHAPTER 13

How to Ease Asthma, Hay Fever, and Emphysema

All sufferers from hay fever and asthma will want to read this chapter carefully. I know what it is to sneeze one's head off and then keep on sneezing and sneezing with never an end in sight. Instead of a handkerchief, I used a sheet. Sometimes I sneezed until I nearly passed out. One day I even set the house on fire because I couldn't see where I put the match after lighting the stove. I was so weak I had fallen down on the bed exhausted. I kept hearing something so I forced myself to go see what it was and there was the kitchen wall in flames. I quickly threw water on it just in time to put it out. So you can see why I am in sympathy with all hay fever sufferers. And I was fast becoming a victim of asthma as well.

How a Child Was Cured of Hay Fever and Asthma

When my husband's eleven-year-old daughter from a distant state came to live with us, she was suffering from hay fever and asthma. We were up with her all of the first night. The reflexes in her hands and feet were too tender for me to work on, and since she didn't know what reflexology was, it upset her more for me to try at that time.

She told us she had been suffering from this chronic disease for five years.

After I explained to her what reflexology was and how it would put an end to her hay fever and asthma attacks, she gladly let me give her a treatment the next day. I started out very gently and worked only a few minutes on her that day, and to our great relief she slept soundly throughout the night.

I kept up the treatments, increasing the pressure and the time of reflex work every day. I also started her on raw honey and honey caps which are excellent for hay fever and asthma, and was careful of her diet. In less than three weeks, she was completely free of all signs of hay fever and asthma and has not had a sign of this distressing disease in twelve years.

HOW TO WORK VARIOUS REFLEXES
FOR RESPIRATORY PROBLEMS

First, let us look at the fingers. We will follow the same procedure that we used for coughs and colds. In the Zone Chart, on page 14, you will see how the middle meridian zone line one runs down the middle of the head, through the nose and on down through the throat, ending on the tips of the thumbs (and big toes). Then on each side of zone one, we have zone two, which also runs down the center of the body, but a little to each side, ending in the tips of the second fingers (and second toes). The same pattern applies to zone three.

Take your thumb in the opposite hand and reflex it, working your thumb and fingers all over it, searching for tender spots. When you find one, you know you are contacting a point of congestion in the corresponding area. So, remember our motto, *If it is sore, work it out.* Work it for a few minutes, and then continue searching for other tender reflexes.

If you find the fingers are not strong enough, or get tired, the reflex comb can be helpful here. Do not forget to press the thumb on the inside next to the index finger as we did in treating coughs. After working the thumb, go on to the index finger and work over it with a press-and-rotate motion. Search out any tender spots, covering the finger on all sides and at the base where it is connected to the hand. Now do the same with the third finger. Also, work the webbing within the Magical V section (between the thumb and index finger). Press-and-roll on the webbing between the second and third fingers, too. Repeat on other hand, searching for tender reflex buttons.

Next, let us use the pressure method. Keeping a steady pressure over the reflexes will achieve excellent results. Using moderately tight pressure, press and hold with the thumb and finger of one hand (or you can use your reflex clamps), on the thumb, second, and third fingers of the opposite hand for ten or fifteen minutes (less, if the fingers start to hurt). Repeat on both hands, several times a day.

Alternatively, you can use the probe-end of your Tongue Cleaning Wand, and press these reflex areas in the center of your tongue, in the same manner that we used it for colds and coughs.

REFLEX HELP FOR ASTHMA ATTACKS

Asthma is an inflammatory disease of the respiratory tract. Mucus production multiplies in the lungs and causes swelling in the airways. This causes coughing and wheezing, and sometimes it is hard to catch a deep breath.

Relaxation is important when an asthma attack begins. When the body relaxes, it minimizes the constriction of the bronchial wall. When the lungs do not receive the oxygen supply they need, the bronchial walls narrow, and this diminishes the air passage.

Learn to recognize what triggers asthma, and its symptoms. As soon as you feel an asthma attack coming on, start calming yourself mentally with a favorite affirmation, prayer, or poem. This intervention will help prevent fear and worry, and can actually be a helpful approach to staying calm.

Relax your mind with calming thoughts: Repeat your favorite covenant, assuring yourself that you can breathe deeply and evenly. Silently tell yourself that you are calm and healthy. Continue this calming meditation while you press the reflex points on the palm of your hand. With a slow and gentle touch, work across the lung and bronchial reflex areas.

Working the left hand first will also include reflex stimulation to the heart, which will help increase circulation and reduce muscular tension, to help you breathe more deeply and freely. Work clear across each hand from the base of fingers, down to the diaphragm and solar plexus points for stress reduction.

CALMING HAY FEVER WITH REFLEXOLOGY

Yes, reflexology has a special message for hay fever suffers, and this holds true for any kind of distress in the respiratory tract. Most treatment for asthma, hay fever, and other infections of the respiratory passages is very similar. Various systems in the body will show improvement under the application of reflexology.

Since we know that hay fever is caused by an allergy, we will treat the whole body to eliminate the underlying cause from malfunctioning glands and organs, especially the ileo-cecal valve (see Chart B, page 11). Lack of calcium is one of the main reasons for allergies of all kinds, according to my good friend, Doctor Smith, D.C., of Roesburg, Oregon.

ADDITIONAL REFLEX HELP FOR UNHEALTHY LUNGS

Let us go over the reflex points that will help diminish asthma trouble. We just learned how important it is to calm your body, so let's press the lung reflex areas on both hands to renew circulation to the lungs and boost up their oxygen supply. Working the lung and bronchial areas, across the upper palm of each hand, can ease breathing and help overcome respiratory problems. While working the reflex areas, inhale a breath of fresh air, hold for five seconds, and then *firmly* exhale for ten seconds to help clear unhealthy air from your lungs.

We have already gone over the throat reflex area on the thumb, and studied the Magical V between the thumb and index finger. I am mentioning it again, as it is so important in helping flush out old toxins that may otherwise form into mucus, and then block the breathing passage. It is especially beneficial if you are coughing.

Also work over both thumbs and the tops of all fingers, encouraging healing energy to the throat, nose, and sinuses passages.

Now work your stomach reflex area to balance energy in the digestive system. (Refer to Chart B, page 11.) Work the reflex areas to both adrenal glands to help the body balance its metabolism. Use the press-and-hold technique as you work the solar plexus and diaphragm reflex in the center of palms to relax nerves and ease breathing.

Place tips of all fingers together and press for seven seconds; release and repeat several times to relax emotional stress (see Photo 17, on page 109). Another method is to fold hands together and squeeze (see Photo 44, on page 257).

Body reflex point:　A pressure point on the body that often helps to calm breathing trouble is the solar plexus and diaphragm body reflex point. Using your index and middle fingers, place them between your breasts and move them down about two inches to the base of the sternum (breastbone). Now take a few deliberate, deep breaths as you slowly press into the reflex area. This may help relax the constricted feeling in the chest, particularly if an asthma attack begins suddenly. Continue pressing this reflex area for a minute or more, with slow, deep breathing. Repeat until the symptoms diminish.

Nourishing foods: Garlic and onions are good for reducing mucus. Drink lots of liquids, including fresh water, apple juice, and cranberry juice, to flush out toxins and enrich your body with the natural power of antiinflammatory vitamins. One tablespoon of fresh lemon juice and honey in hot water helps clear mucus, or put one tablespoon raw apple cider vinegar in a glass of cold water and drink with your meals, to help fight off germs. Eat hot potato and vegetable soup and fresh bananas as they are both high in potassium, which is known to help keep the nerves calm. Stay away from dairy products, fried foods, and sweets, as they may cause mucus.

Supplements for respiratory troubles: Magnesium is given intravenously to treat severe asthma attacks in hospitals and emergency centers. Doctors tell us that magnesium helps relax tiny muscles in the lung airways, which help make breathing easier. Another helpful herb is Ginkgo Biloba—the Chinese have used it for years to treat chronic lung disorders. The extra-potent supplement Ester-C with bioflavonoids quickly carries nutrients into the system, is nonacidic, and circulates through the blood twice as fast as ordinary Vitamin C. Moreover, it is very gentle to the body, and is known to support the natural defense system of the body and promote healthy corrective tissues.

How Reflexology Cures Bronchial Asthma

"Some of the cures of asthma have been little short of miraculous," says Dr. Bowers. "One patient suffering with bronchial asthma had been unable to lie down for three years; what little sleep she did get was when she propped herself up in a chair. Her sole relief consisted in the hypodermic injection of adrenalin solution, practically every morning and night. I made pressure on the tongue with the probe and also on the floor of the mouth directly beneath the root of the tongue.

"Within five minutes this lady—for the first time in three years—was relieved of all pain, tightness, hoarseness, and shortness of breath. In two months of this treatment, she gained fifteen pounds and now sleeps through the night, and she has been able to discontinue completely her use of adrenalin."

Man Reopens Business after Reflexology Cures Asthma

"Another bronchial asthmatic suffered so severely that he had made all arrangements to retire from business and seek health on the Riviera or in Egypt. His wheezing was so pronounced that he could be heard clear across a twenty-foot room. He was advised by Dr. D. F. Sullivan, Senior Surgeon of St. Francis Hospital, to see me before leaving the country.

"I pressed on the floor of the patient's mouth, under the root of the tongue, with a probe and also made strong pressure on the first and second zones of the tongue. In three or four treatments, this man was entirely well, and informed us that he was postponing his trip abroad, and was going back into business again."

REFLEX HELP FOR TUBERCULOSIS AND EMPHYSEMA

Since these are both deteriorating diseases of the respiratory channels, you should treat them in a similar manner when helping nature in her efforts to reactivate the cells back into a healthy condition.

You will, of course, concentrate on the reflexes to the lung that is infected, but not neglecting reflexes to the other lung. All of the reflexes in the fingers should be worked on the sides, as well as the back and palm side. Using a press-and-roll motion, cover all fingers in this manner, and also the webbing between the fingers. After the first two weeks you may work the fingers in this way as often as you like.

To help nature heal this distressing disease, you will want to stimulate the whole body, so work on all of the reflexes in both hands.

The thumb is pressed into the pad lying under the fingers which is the reflex to the lungs, as explained on page 86. Use the pressing rolling motion as you work along this whole area. Now using the same method, work your thumb over the rest of the hand being sure to cover all of the reflexes, even those extending down into the wrists.

If your thumbs and fingers are weak, or become tired too quickly, you can make good use of the Magic Reflexer to help you stimulate the healing forces of nature by reviving electrical activity into all parts of your body. Remember in any deteriorating disease, every cell in your body needs to be brought back up to perfection, not just the part that is in malfunction.

Remember to use a steady pressure to anesthetize or deaden pain, and a rotating method to stimulate and heal.

Emphysema Victim Takes First Deep Breath in Twenty Years

Jean came to me several years ago suffering from an ailment to which the doctors could give no name. She was a very sick woman with no hope of ever recovering when she walked into my office. "I know you cannot help me," she said, "but to please my neighbors and my husband I am here." As I went over the reflexes, I found all of them extremely tender; her whole body was out of harmony, every gland and organ was in discord. Her hands and feet were like ice, but as I worked them, they started to get warm and pink. Jean was amazed. Even though the treatment was very painful, she did not want me to quit. She said she felt like she was coming alive all over. Jean had such a quick and miraculous recovery from her reflex sessions, she wanted to learn how to give this healing regimen to help others back to health. So I suggested she take my course, which she did.

Recently, Jean came to see me, telling of the wonderful success she is having in applying this invigorating therapy on her friends and relatives.

"Nearly everyone laughs when I mention reflexology, they consent to a treatment but with doubts." Then, she says, "they are quite surprised at the results.

"I gave a treatment to my 77-year-old uncle who has had emphysema for years and could hardly breathe. After the treatment, he was able to take his first deep breath in twenty years."

How to Cure
a Sick Voice
with Reflexology

We will all agree that a sick voice is one of the most frustrating things that can happen. We don't realize how much we talk until our voice suddenly becomes silent. Sometimes people suffer for several weeks from laryngitis—barely able to speak above a whisper—not knowing that all they had to do was apply a few minutes of reflex pressure on the fingers and the tongue to get almost immediate and lasting relief.

The technique of working reflexes in the tongue has many benefits in certain instances, which involve zone one, as mentioned in other chapters.

Let us first work reflexes in the hands. We usually work on both hands when stimulating the areas of the throat. This is because the voice box is centralized and would be in zone one, with zones two and three being close enough to give radiations of healing to a lesser degree. (See Charts A and B, pages 10 and 11.)

Take the left thumb and use it to press along the right thumb, on the side next to the right index finger. You can also use your second and third fingers to press this area of the thumb. Notice in Photos 16a and 16b that the index fingers are pressed into the inner side of the thumb, which is definitely a reflex to the voice, in the vocal cord zone.

Keep searching in this area for a sharp sore spot, and when you find it, reflex it for a few seconds, then change hands and search out the tender reflex on your opposite thumb, using the same technique. Now work over both thumbs in the same manner, one at a time. Concentrate on the tender reflex points.

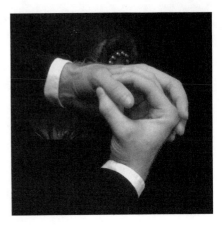

Photo 16a: Press inner-base of
thumb with tip of right index finger.

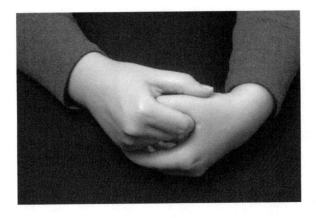

Photo 16b: Position
for pressing the
inner-base of thumb
with inside edge of
folded index finger.

USE TONGUE REFLEXOLOGY
TO EASE THROAT TENSION

Now we come to the technique of stimulating the reflexes in the
tongue. As explained in Chapter 9, you will take a clean cloth and
place it around the tongue; now take it between the thumb and fingers and gently pull it out as far as comfortable, then wiggle it from
side to side. This will relieve a "tight," inflexible throat, which is the
bane of all vocalists and speakers. This method, for instance, was used
for many years by the gifted Italian tenor, Umberto Sorrentino. He
says, "This method eases up throat tension, and frees the voice, and
will abort a cold."

Reflexology Used by Opera Singer to Keep Voice Beautiful

Miss Mabel Garrison, a lyric soprano of the Metropolitan Opera House, also used this method of reflexology not only on herself, but has won the appreciation and gratitude of various members of the company, by curing their stiff, inelastic sore throats.

It is a significant fact that no singer, parent, actor, clergyman, doctor, lawyer or Indian chief can afford to ignore the simple application of reflexology when the voice is affected.

Grandmothers Used Reflexology to Relieve Choking in Croup

Another procedure that can help ease an ailing voice is the probe method on the reflexes in the tongue. In case of coughing and choking, as in croup, our grandmothers knew how to relieve this distress by putting pressure on back of the tongue for a few minutes until the coughing stopped.

MANY SPEAKERS TURN TO REFLEXOLOGY FOR RELIEF OF VOCAL STRAIN

Reflexology has, in numerable instances, restored lost speaking voices. It is a common occurrence to have a clergyman, a lawyer, and other spokespersons who have become voiceless from speeches and long dictation, or some other vocal strain, go to a reflexologist. I have helped those who were unable to speak above a whisper, and within a half hour, they go their way victoriously.

How a Speaker Regained His Voice

It is remarkable what finger pressure alone will accomplish. Mr. A., a politician, had been speaking most of the day at a convention held in an outside grove. The amplifier refused to work so he talked without it. The leafy bowers and mossy dells were not built for acoustic purposes and the consequence was that when darkness closed in, Mr. A. could not speak above a whisper. He had such a contraction of the muscles that he couldn't even open his jaws—let alone talk.

When he presented himself at the office of a reflexologist the next day, he could not open his mouth. It was impossible to treat the reflexes in the tongue, so he was given a durable comb and told to press its teeth on the reflexes in his hands, starting with the end of the thumb and working along to the wrist; also around the first and second fingers covering the whole area. He continued pressing both on the palm, and the back side of the hand, including the webs. He was left to his own devices for about twenty minutes. At the end of this time, tension of the jaw muscles had relaxed, and he had also relieved the irritation in his throat. A tongue depressor was then used, and three days later he was able to resume his speaking.

TECHNIQUE OF FINDING REFLEXES IN THE TONGUE

To use this same technique, it is better to use the clean handle of a table knife, or a spoon handle, if you do not have a tongue probe to press down on the reflexes on the back of the tongue. Sterilize any object before putting it into the mouth.

In case of emergency, the finger can be used, of course. Just place whatever tool is being used in the back part of the mouth without making yourself gag. Press down on the tongue, searching for tender spots here as you would on the fingers. When you find a tender spot, hold the pressure on it for a few seconds or minutes, according to the condition of your throat. The handles of the Stirling Tongue Wand convert into a probe, often used to press the reflexes in the tongue. (See Photo 65, page 286.)

Almost everyone suffers occasionally from defects somewhere in the delicate mechanism that shapes the air currents into beautiful sounds, and molds the breath into speech or song.

Professional Performers Helped by Reflexology

In other arts such as ballet, theater, etc., where performers must remain at the peak of talent at all times, reflexology treatments have helped in many ways: better breath control, fewer colds, and relaxation from tension both muscular and of the nervous system, which are a threat to performance. These treatments resulted in greater confidence and less anxiety.

An important voice teacher in the city often sent students to reflexologist Mrs. Roon to give help in these areas. Mrs. Roon had been a professional singer herself and understood well what the problems could be and how to help them with reflexology. She was a dear person, full of projects and activities and always glad to be of help. When singers left her office, they were soon feeling healthy and ready to perform.

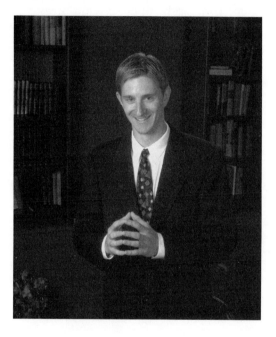

Photo 17: Relieving tension by pressing tips of fingers together.

HOW TO RELAX WHILE MAKING A SPEECH

My son-in-law tells me of an experience he had with reflexology before realizing what he was doing.

He had to give a talk to a group of salespeople and, not being practiced at making speeches, he was quite nervous. He said he was so upset when he first got up in front of the group that he couldn't even think of the speech he had practiced beforehand. In his nervousness, he unconsciously pressed the tips of his fingers together as he talked and suddenly he felt relaxed, and at ease, as he continued his talk, finishing it with great success. But he remembers that he kept the tips of his fingers pressed tightly together all through the talk.

Now he realizes that it was the act of pressing the fingers together that brought him relaxation at the high point of tension and made it possible to feel at ease through the rest of his speech. But at the time he was not aware of using one of nature's powerful forces to relaxing his nerves.

Press the tips of all your fingers together as in Photo 17 on page 109. Use a slight pressure for a few moments and feel the surge of electric currents vibrating through your body.

CHAPTER 15

How Reflexology Can Stop Your Headache

Here is an example of how headache pain can be "pressed" out. A typical case reported by Dr. George Starr White may be helpful.

A lady suffered from a severe headache on the top of her head, which had persisted for more than three weeks. She had consulted several doctors who had given her drugs and hypodermics, but the relief was only temporary.

Dr. White told her nothing of what was contemplated, but took hold of her hands and began firmly pressing on the first, second, and third fingers—the pain being diffused over the frontal regions—at the same time engaging her in conversation concerning her condition. After about three minutes, he asked her if she could indicate with her hand just where the pain was.

She hesitated, looked up, and said, "Do you use mental therapy?" Then, after blinking perplexedly for half a minute, she added, "For the first time in three weeks, except when I've been under the influence of narcotics, the pain is entirely gone." Dr. White told her to have someone repeat these finger pressures, at the same time emphasizing that if she failed to get relief from this method, to come back. He has not seen her since.

Remember that the same condition may not clear up from the same point every time, even in the same patient. At one time, we might stop pain by pressing the forefinger, and another time the point would be found some place on the thumb, or the middle finger, or even in the webbing between fingers.

Always work the pad in both thumbs, a reflex that corresponds to the brain. Promoting stimulation to the brain will help release a pain-killing substance called endorphins, which is a natural substance that suppresses pain. (See Photo 4 on page 30, Photo 22a on page 132, and photo 51 on page 280).

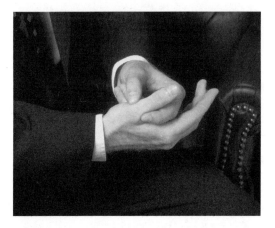

Photo 18: Position for working reflexes around the base of the right thumb.

REFLEX HELP FOR VARIOUS TYPES OF HEADACHE PAIN

First, you will work the reflexes around both thumbs, as these correspond to your head and neck. Now take each thumb, one at a time, and give it two or three light twists and rolls for relaxing. Also, inhale several deep breaths to take in oxygen. This will help unlock internal energy, which the head needs to clear away pain.

Pinched nerves: A pinched nerve in the neck or spine can cause a headache. In this case, we will work on the thumb, working up and down the spinal reflex area (see Chart B, page 11). Concentrate on reflexes along the upper edge of your thumb, as they correspond to the upper part of your neck, "the cervical spine."

Tension headaches: A tension headache can be brought on from tight muscles in the neck. After you have given the thumb a good workout, take it between the thumb and first two fingers of the opposite hand, and start to roll it—first to the right and then to the left, around and around several times each way. Repeat on the other thumb. Soon you will find yourself relaxing. This gives the same relaxing sensation that you would get if someone took your head in their hands and gently rolled it around and around, from side to side.

Letters come to us from people all over the world, telling of the wonderful results they had in stopping their headaches after following directions in my book *Foot Reflexology*. On the foot, you can roll and rotate the big toe, which corresponds to the neck reflexes, same as with the thumb. Then you can follow right on down the foot on the spine reflexes. Again, it will be the same on the hand.

Reflexology reduces stress in the neck, which relaxes muscles that could be causing a tension headache. First work the thumb in zone one, then move to the index finger next to it, in zone two. Between them, at the basal joints are special reflexes that stop many colds, headaches, and help calm stress.

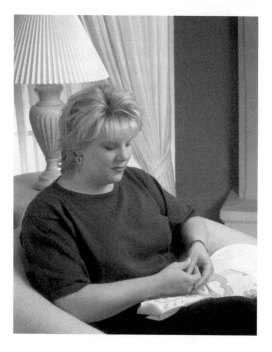

Photo 19: Position for working reflexes in the left thumb to relieve tension and headache pain from the left side of neck.

The stomach: In many cases, the stomach is the cause of headaches. If finger pressure on the thumb does not stop the head pain within a few minutes, then try the reflexes to the stomach (see Chart B, page 11). The reflexes to the stomach will be found near the magical V webbing, between the thumb and index finger, also slightly over into the center of the hand a bit. When reflexing the Magical V section, you are sending healing energy to both the head and stomach at the same time. (See Photo 7, page 33).

Constipation could be the problem. Work across the stomach reflex with the rolling, pressing motion learned earlier in the book. Be careful in working this area for very long if you have an upset or weak stomach, as it might make you nauseated. However, do not let this stop you from working the stomach reflexes, as the stimulation will give you a healthy, strong stomach in time. So, keep at it, slowly at first. Also work the entire reflex area to the large and small intestine across both hands (see Illustration 18, page 158). Once constipation is no longer the problem, you will be amazed at how quickly you will forget that you ever had a stomachache or a headache.

Sinus headaches: Blocked sinuses are a painful situation, sometimes affecting only one side of the head, sometimes the eyes, and other times the whole head. If you suffer from sinus trouble, work the tips of all fingers and both thumbs. (See Photo 3, page 29.) Also, work the webbing between all fingers to help open up sinuses within the corresponding zones. I always work up and down each finger and both thumbs, as well.

Body reflex pressure is very beneficial during a sinus attack. Placing a rotating pressure on your face where it hurts, over the eye, or on the temple will often help break up sinus congestion, and free a natural flow of circulation to the painful area, thus stopping a sinus headache. Pinching the eyebrows, and between the eyes over your nose, may also help release painful sinus congestion.

Eyestrain or cluster headaches: Pain can be brought on by a weak kidney or from nervous tension. To dispel pain with reflexology, work the reflex buttons to calm the nerves, along all fingers, including the thumb, on the same side as the pain. In addition, press and hold on the solar plexus reflex in the center of each palm, as this corresponds to a system of nerves within the center of the body. Relaxing this system can relax the whole body.

For eyestrain, work the eye reflex area, where the fingers meet your palm, and the webbing between the second and third fingers, as well as the reflexes around the base of these two fingers.

Refer to Chart B (page 11) for location of kidney reflex. Search for a tender spot and work it with a press-and-rotate motion for a few seconds, then return to it later and give it another workout. Read more about the kidneys in Chapter 29. Once you have worked the soreness out, the kidney will most likely be well and the headaches will stop.

Helpful tips: Turn down the lights, and move away from computers and work stations with bright lights, or disturbing glares. Relax your eyes with a few eye exercises. Work the eye muscles by looking far away, then looking at something close by. Next, roll your eyes clockwise and then counterclockwise one or two times. Do not overdo.

Prevention is important: Make sure to wear your sunglasses when you go outside. Excessive sunlight can cause squinting, as well as strained facial and neck muscles. It can also cause a severe headache.

Migraines: Poor circulation to the brain, food allergies, or severe body tension can lead to migraines. Work all reflexes in the fingers to relax nerves and reduce stress. Work the spine and head reflex areas to increase circulation to the brain. Reflex the pituitary gland in the pads of your thumbs and all other endocrine glands to balance hormones and release endorphins. Always work both hands. Work the lungs and heart reflex, across both hands, to encourage circulation of blood and oxygen throughout the body and to the head.

Work the liver reflex to encourage the elimination of toxins, and to help improve your digestion and metabolism. The liver plays an important role in the health of your whole body, and when it is not working smoothly can cause a severe migraine. Work this organ reflex thoroughly, yet gently on the right hand or right foot.

Poor circulation can also cause headaches, so work the reflexes in your hands and fingers, and rub your hands together to get the circulation moving. Bend your hands at the wrists, and your feet at the ankles. The Deluxe Hand & Foot Roller is very helpful for stimulating circulation through the hands and feet. (See Photo 32, page 196, and Photo 46, page 261.) This revitalizing invigoration helps move currents of healing energy throughout the entire body, even to the head.

How Reflexology Helped a Square Dancer

My husband and I were at a square dance festival a few days ago when some very good friends came up to tell us good-bye. Since it was early in the evening, we asked why they were leaving before the dance was over. The couple explained that the man had a terrible headache. I had noticed that he had been quite list-less earlier in the evening.

My husband showed him how to press the top (or back) of the thumb with the thumb of the opposite hand until he found a ten-der place. He told him then to continue to work it for a few min-utes, or until the headache was better.

We thought they had gone home until we saw them later. They were dancing and his eyes looked bright and free from pain. They danced the rest of the evening, even joining the crowd for dinner later. He said he felt completely free from his headache, thanks to the thumb massage, even if it was hard to believe. He told us later that the headaches had been frequent for years, but now he knew how to stop them, and even prevent them from starting. He was very grateful.

SPREAD THE NEWS OF REFLEXOLOGY

It would indeed be a marvelous sum total of health, happiness, and economic efficiency if all headaches, for instance, would be cured, and kept cured, by reflexology.

Many appreciative people are spreading the knowledge of this wonderful technique of simply working the fingers and toes, to do away with the need of resorting to dangerous drugs! We must carry this teaching to its only logical conclusion and teach others how to use this perfectly safe and harmless way to health. People may, if sick, cure themselves of their minor ailments! If your doctor can't help you, why not try reflexology? It is safe! And everyone receives some benefit.

How a Hangover Was Quickly Relieved

Reflexology will even relieve headache from a hangover. My hus-band was with a fishing party where some of the men spent one evening drinking. One of the men complained of a terrible headache the next morning. Nothing he took seemed to bring relief. My hus-band told him to rub his thumb with the opposite thumb and forefin-ger. He looked skeptical, but being in pain, he tried it, and was amazed that his headache was gone almost instantly. He went around telling everyone about it. And he said he felt great, too—no more hangover!

The next time you have a headache, instead of attempting to paralyze the nerves of sensation with an opiate or pain deadener, try working the reflexes in your thumb. You will find it rather tender at first but keep massaging it a few minutes and feel the wonderful relief as the pain lifts from you.

If the headache is in the middle of the head, working the thumb reflex will usually stop it in a very few minutes, and in many cases almost immediately.

I have received many letters telling of the success of those who have used this method to stop their headaches with nothing else but working their big toes! But in many cases it is easier and more convenient to work the thumb. This can be done even in public without being noticed by anyone. You will find that it also relieves nervousness.

How Reflexology Changed My Life

Your book *Helping Yourself with Foot Reflexology* has changed my life. Would you believe that I cured myself of lifelong headaches within three minutes by following your directions? And as an added bonus I cured myself of chronic canker sores at the very same time. I mean to tell you that canker sores healed up at once, immediately, the very same day as my headaches were cured.

The very first night I slept completely through the night, never getting up once to go to the bathroom. All this happened to me the very first day. Unbelievable but true. Thanks to you.

You will be happy to learn that two of our friends were cured of hemorrhoids within three weeks. Two other friends were cured of prostate trouble within three days. They followed the directions in your book.

We are so indebted to you, Mrs. Carter, and the only way I can repay you is to tell all of our friends and relatives of your wonderful book.

Thank you and kindest regards.

Sincerely and gratefully yours,

J.P., California

A Doctor Chiro-Podiatrist Has Success with Reflexology

I am getting some good results with a few patients and friends of mine. Would like to know if there is anyone doing reflexology work in this area. I have people I could refer to them for treatments. I find the book very interesting and helpful.

Sincerely,

A.D.D., D.S.C.

Reflexology Is a True Blessing

Dear Ms. Carter,

I have read and reread your wonderful book and have decided to make reflexology my life's work. I have used the techniques of reflex body massage on my entire family and everyone has benefited from it. My (soon to be) daughter-in-law has suffered from terrible migraine headaches. The only thing she found that would help at all is very potent medication in the form of a shot that her doctor would administer, and which she eventually learned to give to herself. These shots totally put her "out" for the entire day, and afterwards she feels groggy and disoriented.

As she was getting one of her headaches, I asked if I could give her a reflexology treatment. I gave her a very thorough treatment and she immediately felt better and said she thought she'd like to lie down awhile. After about an hour's nap she was up and said she had no sign of a headache.

I have since taught my son how to give her a reflexology treatment and he does this whenever she feels a headache coming on. It's been a true blessing. I have helped my mother, brother, sister, and my oldest son with various ailments and they can hardly believe the results. Thank you for sharing this wonderful form of alternative medicine.

Sincerely,

D. J. S., Missouri

CHAPTER 16

How to Stop Hair Loss with Reflexology

A beautiful frame brings to life even the dullest of pictures.

Your hair is the frame for your face and its beauty or lack of beauty makes the difference in how you look to the world. Baldness used to confine itself mostly to men, but today women put their hair under so much stress from the use of chemicals for permanents, dyes, and so on, that they are taking their place along with the balding men.

HAIR IS BAROMETER OF YOUR HEALTH

Hair, like the nails, is a modified skin structure similar to the outer layer of the skin. The hair is peculiarly sensitive to the condition of the health of the body. If, for any cause, the system is depleted, it shows in the hair before any other place.

Scientists tell us to take protein, silica, and calcium for beautiful hair and strong, beautiful fingernails; yet, no one has mentioned the vital electrical force activating stimulation between the hair and nails. Both the hair and nails are made of the same substance and are cut at regular intervals. They are on the same electrical current of healing forces waiting for the right button to be pushed to help nature revive glandular activity.

Doctor Gives Magic Secret of How to Grow New Hair

I am going to tell you the secret, told by the late Dr. Joe Shelby Riley, that will not only stop your falling hair, but will help you grow

119

a new head of hair successfully. If you are combing your hair out by the handfuls, then you will be forever grateful for yet another of nature's simple techniques of using reflexology not only to free you from the embarrassment of hair loss, but also to help you grow a beautiful new head of hair even if you are now bald. Here is the Magic Secret:

Rub the fingernails of one hand directly across the fingernails of the other hand with a quick, rapid motion as though you were buffing them with a buffer, only you are using the fingernails of the opposite hand as the buffer. Do this for five minutes at least three times a day.

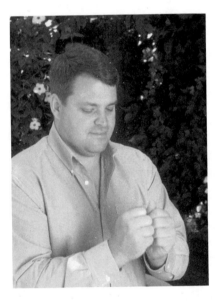

Photo 20: Position for buffing fingernails to stimulate the regrowth of hair.

How to Use Reflexology to Prevent Gray Hair

This miracle of new hair won't happen in a day or two. You must keep at it. The first thing you will notice in a few weeks is that the hair has stopped falling out. If you are young, that is, before your hair has begun to turn gray, and you do this for five minutes, night and morning, you will build up the entire nerve force of your body.

As nerve force is the foundation of a perfect organ, stimulate the hair molecules into life and you will have plenty of hair as long as you live and will never have a gray hair the rest of your life. Thousands of people 60 and 70 years of age who have been doing this all their lives are living witness to the truth of this statement. Concentrate on this as you do it. Don't let up. Keep in mind what you wish to accomplish.

This magic secret of stimulating the reflexes in the fingernails will be a boon, not only to balding men and women, but to those who have discovered that first gray hair.

Previously Bald Author Has Luxurious Hair at Seventy

Dr. Riley, the author of this system was bald, and he said, as many others have said,

> "Oh, it is natural to be bald. My father was bald and my grand-father was bald before he was forty. I quit wearing a hat and started to use the exercises as described above, and soon my head began to have a fuzz, and then the hair began to grow, and now at over seventy years of age I have a fine luxurious head of hair."

Woman's Hair Changes from Gray to Blonde

A lovely woman named Grace wrote a letter saying she wanted to improve her state of health, so she started using reflexology on her hands, feet, and body. She even buffed her fingernails everyday. She wrote that her health had greatly improved since using the reflex therapy, and that something else very unexpected transpired. Her salt-and-pepper hair was growing out its original color, a beautiful golden blonde, as when she was younger. Further, she sent the cutest videotape of herself to prove it.

Buff your nails and work the reflexes to your endocrine glands to charge up the natural hormonal balance for better hair growth. Many thousands who have used these secret methods of reflexology now rejoice because of the beautiful head of hair that frames their faces. Reread Dr. Riley's Magic Secret—then, "Go thou and do likewise." Give nature a chance.

CHAPTER 17

Anemia Can Be Helped with Reflexology

Anemia is a condition where there is not enough oxygen carried to the cells and a lack of iron in the bloodstream. When people have anemia, they may feel weak, fatigued, dizzy, have pale gums and fingernails, and have a hard time breathing, although they have not been physically active. The spleen serves as a storehouse for iron needed by the blood. If neglected for a long period, anemia can cause serious health troubles.

If you will look at Charts A and B (pages 10 and 11), you will see how the spleen is located on the left side of the body down from the heart. The reflex to the spleen and heart are on the left hand. If you are anemic, you will have no trouble finding a tender spot in the spleen reflex. This may be a small spot, about the size of a pea. If it is sore, use your thumb to press and rotate on this button until you have worked the soreness out. You will be helping nature stimulate this congested gland from being lazy, back into a healthy condition.

ANEMIA DRAINS ENERGY

When I was very young, a doctor told me I was so anemic I had the energy of an eighty-year-old woman. I was so tired it was an effort for me to get out of bed, let alone walk around. If you ever feel like that, work the spleen reflex to see if you can find any tenderness. When you do, work it out.

Remember how important the liver is to the entire body. Work the liver reflex area on the right hand, or foot, to relieve physical weakness, and help the body eliminate toxins, as well as improve digestion and promote the absorption of iron into the blood-stream.

Remember that the spleen is the storage container of your life-energy forces. So, keep it in perfect condition by working its reflexes, along with those of the heart, lungs, and liver to help protect and reserve rich red blood cells.

Anemia may also be due to a Vitamin B_{12}, iron, or folic acid deficiency. White spots may appear under fingernails when your system is anemic. Some iron-rich foods are figs, molasses, beets, raisins, prunes, yams, almonds, whole grains, seafood, and dark greens.

How a Man Regained Energy

About three weeks ago I became run down, no pep, no usual get-up-and-go. I had been reading about the spleen in your book on Foot Reflexology. I thought maybe that could be my trouble.

Sure enough, the spleen reflex was very sore—so I massaged it, first day about a minute, next day a little longer. After about three days, I was my usual self. Sounds like a fairy story, but it *really worked*. Now I massage my own feet every day. Thanks to Mrs. Carter, I feel great.

Mr. B. R.

Dramatic Improvement in Energy Level

I have been using reflexology faithfully for six months and I notice a dramatic improvement in my energy level. It has helped me feel better and increased my productivity at work. I used to drag home, eat, and go to bed. Instead now, I feel great stamina all day long and actually have extra energy after work. Today I even participate in varied evening activities at the community center.

Thank you for all your marvelous teachings!

D.N.

Dear Mrs. Carter:

I have already experienced a change in my body since buying your book *Helping Yourself with Foot Reflexology.* I used to be tired all the time. Now hardly ever so. I know it works.

Mrs. A.N.N.

How to Treat Arthritis with Reflexology

Arthritis is an updated name for rheumatism, which has caused suffering throughout the ages. We now know that it attacks in many forms. There are over a hundred different kinds of arthritis. The most common are rheumatoid arthritis, osteoarthritis, gout, and systemic lupus erythematosus. Each type has a different target area. Some affect the joints, others the tendons. Some arthritis sufferers have tender muscles, others have articular or painful joints. Arthritic disease causes painful, disabling symptoms and suffering to millions of Americans.

There are several things that you can do at home to help manage your own care. Reflexology and exercise help to relieve arthritis at all stages, and are key factors for increasing circulation and flexibility to affected joints. Controlling stress, exercising as able, and eating whole foods are also helpful ways to heal arthritis.

The body is a wonderful work of art that no man can duplicate. It takes years and years of abuse and neglect to bring about the eventual breakdown of this intricate wonder. Then people question why they start having aches and pains when they should be at the very peak of health. "Just when I could start enjoying life," they say, "this had to happen to me."

Fortunately, however, we can treat arthritis at any stage with reflexology, restoring lost functioning, alleviating aches and pains, and halting further damage to one's system. Reflexology is a valuable therapy for arthritis sufferers because it helps balance the internal organs by revitalizing circulation. This renewed stimulation helps flush out organic wastes and toxins, such as salt deposits and uric acid, that would otherwise promote inflammation and sore joints in the body.

A recent study at Stanford University showed a dramatic difference after patients used self-help measures. They soon had increased flexibility, improved strength, and better endurance. The Arthritis Foundation reported the patients even reduced their doctor visits by 43 percent.

Reflexology has helped many arthritis sufferers control the negative effects of swelling and pain. You, too, can help yourself fight arthritis and reduce pain without side effects from drugs or serious complications from surgical procedures.

HOW ARTHRITIS AFFECTS THE WHOLE BODY

The most serious form of arthritis is called *rheumatoid arthritis*. It is extremely painful and a crippling disease that affects people of all ages, particularly young adults. Women are afflicted with rheumatoid arthritis three times more often than men.

Paavo O. Airola, N.C., writes in his book *There Is a Cure for Arthritis:*

> It is important to realize that although swollen and inflamed joints may seem to be the very first signals of approaching arthritis, they are not at all the first symptoms of the onset of the disease. Arthritis is not a local disease of a particular joint but a systemic disorder, a disease which affects the entire body.
>
> The arthritis patient usually suffers from a general deterioration of health in the form of sluggishness in the function of his vital organs; incomplete digestion and assimilation of food; nutritional deficiencies; glandular disorders, *particularly in the endocrine system;* impaired elimination of metabolic wastes and toxins; and a weakened nervous system and circulation. These systemic disturbances affect the biochemical structure of the various tissues of the body and cause what one of the pioneer practitioners of biological medicine in the United States, R. P. Watterson, M.D., calls a "biochemical suffocation."

HOW YOU CAN RELIEVE ARTHRITIS

When using reflexology, we are opening the channels in all parts of the body and we can readily see why people are having such wonderful results when they use reflexology to help arthritis. Every time a reflex button is pressed, it instantly sends a charge of magnetic vital life force surging through the body to the particular area with which it is in contact, opening and stimulating the pathway as it goes.

When you press many reflex buttons, you can picture what is happening all through your body's network of intricate channels. No wonder you feel so exhilarated with renewed life and vitality immediately after a reflex workout! You have released the clogged channels, leaving no place of biochemical suffocation.

REACTIVATE GLANDULAR SYSTEM TO EASE PAIN

First you should concentrate on activating the endocrine glands, and then follow through by working the rest of the glands and organs until you have covered all the reflexes, to every part of your body.

The importance of the endocrine system: Once we realize that our glandular system is the transmitter of life forces that are transformed into function through the body, we can readily understand the importance of using reflexology. This will stimulate the transmission pattern of the electrical network of the body.

So, let us take a quick look at the Endocrine Chart on page 57. Notice how the glands are located near the center of the head and body. You can see then why we concentrate our reflex work on the first, second, and third zones of the fingers and hands.

Working the pituitary gland reflex: Since the pituitary is the king gland, you should start working the center of the pad on the thumb as shown in Photo 4, page 30 and Photo 51, page 280. Then move on to the pineal and hypothalamus reflexes, which are located just a little toward the side of the thumb. When you work the reflexes in the pad of both thumbs, you will be stimulating all three glands.

You may work these reflex buttons either with the rolling-and-pressing motion or by holding solid pressure on them. You can do this with the working edge of the thumb, or the tip of your index finger, using the opposite hand. Alternatively, you can hold a steady pressure on the reflex with a clamp. Clamps can be held for a longer period of time and used on several fingers at once.

Working the thyroid, parathyroid, and thymus glands: To stimulate these important glands, we press into reflexes around the base of the thumb, using the thumb of your opposite hand or the Magic Reflexer.

Working the pancreas and adrenal glands: Let us look at the pancreas on the Endocrine Chart (page 30) to see how it lies in front of the adrenal glands. Since the reflexes to these glands are so close together, you can work them at the same time. Press the thumb into the reflex area using a rolling, pressing motion. These reflexes may be more sensitive than most of the others, so you will not need a hard pressure here. The Magic Reflexer will cover these reflexes quite satisfactorily if you have one.

Keep in mind that the reflexes in the palm are going to activate the more sensitive organs and glands in your body, *so you must not over-work them for the first two weeks.* Work the reflex to these glands, two or three minutes on each hand, every other day for the first week.

Reactivating your reproductive system: Now we move to the gonads, which are the ovaries in women and the testes in men. These are the organs of reproduction, but they also produce hormones that create the inner warmth in our system, preventing all tendencies for inflexibility, hardening, and stiffening. No wonder they play such an important part in arresting the development of arthritis!

You will notice on your chart that the reflexes to these all-important glands are located on the lower part of the hand and into the wrist area. To give reflexes to these glands the proper amount of work, use the thumb of the opposite hand and work the whole area of the wrist, starting under the little finger and working over to the center of the wrist. If you hold your hand up with the back toward you, this would be the outside of the hand, the same as the outside of the foot on which these glands are located under the ankle.

FLUSH OUT CLOGGED CHANNELS

Stimulate the liver: Now that you have activated all the endocrine glands, let us look at the reflex to the liver and a few other organs that will help flush toxic wastes from the body. You will find the liver reflex in your right hand (see Photo 35, page 213). Place the thumb of your left hand on your right palm; start on the little finger side of your hand, using the press-and-rotate, or the walking motion, to work across your hand. Move your thumb down a bit, and work back across the hand until you have covered the entire liver reflex area. Also work the webbing between the thumb and index finger, working on any tender buttons you may find there.

Working reflexes to the lungs, heart, kidneys, and stomach: Let us go to the area under the fingers and across the right hand first. Work this whole area into the pad that lies in the upper third of the palm, where the lung reflex is located.

Now work across the left hand to stimulate energy to the left lung and the heart. This will help renew the movement of oxygen and blood throughout the systems. Improved circulation means a better supply of oxygen and nutrients.

Stimulate the kidney reflex in both hands to help remove excess acids from your body. Then work the reflex to the stomach, across the left palm.

Diet is important to healing arthritis: Drink a lot of juice and eat raw fruits and vegetables, leafy greens, garlic, onions, oats, eggs, whole grains, fish, raisins, prunes, and blackstrap molasses. Foods to avoid are tomatoes, green peppers, potatoes, fatty foods, sugar, eggplant, and spicy foods. They have an acidic substance to which arthritis sufferers seem to be very pain-sensitive.

Work all reflexes in both hands: Do not forget to search for tender buttons in the webbing between all fingers. Also, keep in mind that by activating just one tiny pinpoint in your reflexes, you can send an electrical charge of vital force into a clogged channel, releasing a kingpin that has been the cause of all your trouble.

A metabolic disorder and systemic disturbances cause arthritis, particularly in glandular activity, which bring about pathological and biochemical changes in all tissues of the body. We can easily understand why so many victims of this dreaded disease are getting such astonishing results when they reactivate the whole glandular system with reflexology.

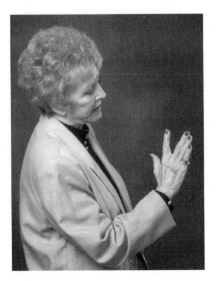

Photo 21: Slightly stretching finger joint allows nourishment to the cells and cartilage. It also helps preserve flexibility.

HOW RENEWED CIRCULATION HELPS STOP PAIN

Working the reflex areas around the thumbs and wrists will encourage lymph to move throughout the body. Waste is removed by the lymphatic system. (If it were left to accumulate within the muscles, they would swell with stagnant fluids and accumulate metabolic buildup that would cause pain and stiffness.)

Lymph is stimulated by the motion of the arms, legs, wrists, and ankles, so move them frequently. Breathing also helps the movement of lymph, so take in long, slow breaths.

Reflexology is a natural prescription for good health, as it helps renew circulation and promotes relaxation, both very important in helping promote the body's own healing powers. Reflex stimulation brings warmth to blood and eases aching muscles and joints.

HOW TO PRESERVE YOUR MUSCLES AND JOINTS

Motion is extremely beneficial to cartilage that covers the ends of joints and bones. If the fluid stagnates around the cartilage that covers them, no nourishment will get to the joints and they will become stiff and sore. So you can see how important it is to keep your joints moving.

Try these exercises to increase flexibility: Gently stretch and bend one finger at a time up and down, and then from side to side.

Another exercise is to stand next to a wall and "walk" your fingers up as high as possible, alternating all fingers, like a spider. Then walk fingers back down the wall again. Reaching up high is beneficial for your shoulders, too. This exercise will help you retain flexibility.

Do exercises that help strengthen your hands, wrists, and fingers. For example, simply squeeze the Magic Reflexer with each hand and then with the thumb and one finger at a time. (See Photo 22 on page 312.)

Good preventative techniques are equally beneficial, such as gently waving good-bye, or moving your hands sideways to the left, then the right.

Rub your hands together and gently work the reflexes to stimulate renewed circulation. Also refer to the hand and finger rotations shown in Illustration 10 on page 25. Also see the backward wrist stretch, Illustration 17, page 139. Practice moving all your joints and muscles to keep them flexible.

A fun and easy way to increase finger strength and flexibility: Press your thumb and one finger at a time against the Magic Reflexer. Repeat exercise with each finger. First press with your thumb and index finger, count to seven, and relax. Repeat three times and then change fingers. Next, press with your thumb and third finger; then thumb and fourth finger; and last but not least, with your thumb and fifth finger.

To strengthen fingers, wrists, and forearms, squeeze the Reflexer hard in each hand for seven seconds, relax, and repeat as necessary.

How a Ranch Woman Recovered from Arthritis

A very kind friend named Annie tries to help everyone she meets, no matter what his or her problems. One day she told me about a neighbor of hers, on an adjoining ranch. Annie watched this woman become ill with arthritis; she noticed it spreading over the body little by little. This woman was becoming helpless, no longer able to even enjoy a walk outside on her ranch.

Visitor from France brings reflexology: Annie tells of the unexpected way in which she was introduced to my book on foot reflexology. The relative of another neighbor, who was visiting from

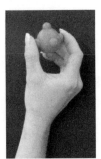

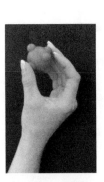

a: Thumb and index finger

b: Thumb and third finger

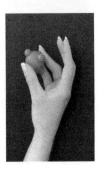

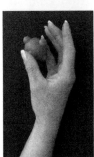

c: Thumb and fourth finger

d: Thumb and little finger

Photo 22: To strengthen fingers, press thumb and one finger at a time against the Magic Reflexer.

France, loaned it to her. Annie enjoyed the book, and immediately sent for one of her own. She started studying it and using the techniques on her feet. Once she felt she knew where the reflexes were located, she went to her neighbor who was afflicted with arthritis and asked if she would like to try reflexology, since it could do no harm.

Annie said that her neighbor seemed to feel improvement the first day she tried the reflex therapy on her. The very first night, the woman slept the whole night through, without waking once.

Anyone familiar with reflexology knows the feeling of relaxation and being able to sleep soundly through the night. It is usually the first sign that the body is receiving benefits from the workout session. Remember, the body heals while we sleep. This is why doctors give drugs to help us sleep. Reflexology, instead of making you feel drugged when you wake up, gives you the feeling of renewed vitality and pep.

Annie tells of the surprisingly quick recovery of her neighbor: "Today she can walk as well as I can. She has resumed her outside work on the ranch with joy, thanks to reflexology!"

The Impossible Becomes Possible

Dear Mrs. Carter,

As long as one has the faith, nothing is impossible. Just take the case of two women patients, both suffering from the crippling disease, Rheumatoid Arthritis. Unbelievable as it may seem, but it's true—Mrs. T. can play tennis, while Mrs. N. can dance again. At first, I thought these would be hopeless cases. But the faith I have in your books gave me the supreme power. This dreadful disease attacked all joints in the body, but most of all, the back portion of the knees. It is hard like a rock. So I applied the body reflexology and deep muscle therapy, with the assistance of the Reflex Massage Board; they recovered in less than six months. Another beauty of reflexology is that these women are able to cut down their medication. Thanks for your chapter on the importance of the endocrine glands. Through that process, I have helped many suffering people.

With best regards,

B.C.

How Reflexology Helps Stop Carpal Tunnel Syndrome and Wrist Pain

Your hands are an important part of your body, and when they hurt, you hurt all over. No one wants to suffer with painful hands. Nevertheless, thousands of people who work or have a hobby that requires repetitious wrist movements find that they are experiencing unpleasant tingling sensations or even dull aches in the wrist, thumb, and middle fingers. When this happens, it is a sign that circulation is slowing in the tiny tunnel space within the wrist.

If not taken care of, other symptoms such as shooting pains and numbness could soon follow. Whether your discomfort is from carpal tunnel syndrome (CTS), arthritis, or just overstressed joints, you will want to release muscle tensions and restore circulation to prevent pain and swelling. One of the first things to do when you notice a wrist problem is to move your hands in a slow, harmonious, circular movement, first to the left and then to the right to release pressure and restore circulation. (See Illustration 10, page 25.)

Hand anatomy: The structure of our hands is very interesting. Each hand has 27 bones. Extending from the wrist to the knuckles are five cylinder-shaped metacarpal bones, and from these metacarpals extend the 14 jointed finger bones.

Eight small cobblestone-shaped bones fit together to bridge the hand and forearm. These are our carpal bones, which make up the wrist. Strong ligaments, tendons, and muscles hold this collection of small bones together (see Illustration 15).

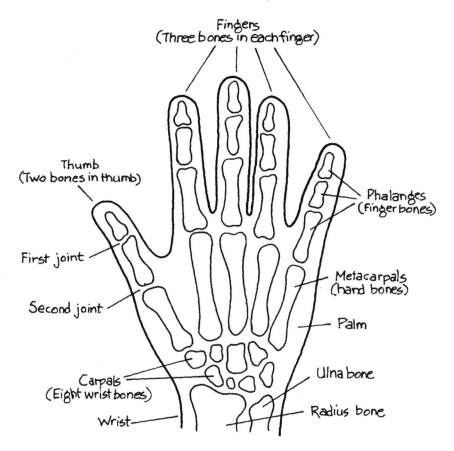

Illustration 15: Bones give our hands their strength. The thumb is opposed to the fingers, which help us pick up objects and do our reflexology work.

TO UNDERSTAND CTS, CREATE YOUR OWN VISUAL AID

First, open your hand with palm facing downward toward the floor. Take your index and fourth fingers, and place them over your middle finger. You can see, by touching them together above your middle finger, how this creates a tunnel effect. The open space symbolizes (in a much-exaggerated way) the tiny hollow gap underneath the ligament of your wrist, which the median nerve passes through. (See Illustration 16.)

When this gap is open, nerve flow is easy and painless. However, when you overuse the wrist, by continually bending or repeating the same motions, the strain on the tunnel structure becomes inflamed. This causes swelling and tormenting pain.

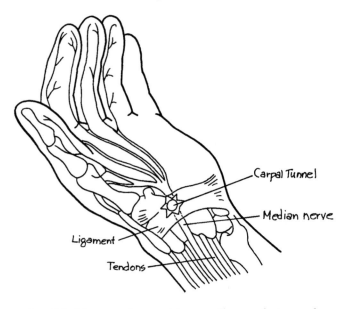

Illustration 16: The carpal tunnel is a small space between bones, ligaments, and tendons in the wrist. Repetitive movements day after day can cause a swelling pressure on the median nerve, producing pain and numbness in the wrist, thumb, and middle finger.

Take a Reflex Break Every Hour

Daily attention with a few good reflexology pressure points and wrist exercises is the best preventative treatment you can give yourself. If you work at a computer, for example, or in a job where your hand is repetitiously moving toward the outside of your body (little finger side), it could be putting pressure on the carpal tunnel. The pressure is squeezing against the median nerve (as it passes through the gap in the front of your wrist) and can cause swelling and inflammation.

For example, our neighbor has a sister who works in a prison. Her job consists of opening cell doors several hours a day. Repetitively twisting keys to the right, toward her little finger, caused her to have CTS.

You can help prevent wrist problems by frequently moving, pressing, and stretching your hands. This, and changing hand positions, will help you avoid conditions such as tenosynovitis (inflammation of a tendon sheath), CTS, and arthritis.

It is a good idea to take a five- or ten-minute break once every hour to move your wrists in the opposite direction from their repetitious movements. Do some reflexology techniques, along with a few hand exercises, to release tension and renew nerve energy through the tunnel. This will also help keep the blood flowing and alleviate pressure on the nerves.

REFLEXOLOGY TECHNIQUES TO EASE WRIST AND HAND PAIN

Release the tension from your hand and wrist by finding the Magical V section between the webbing of your thumb and index finger. Use the press-and-rotate technique for a few minutes on this reflex area to stimulate healing circulation through the energy zone to the carpal tunnel within the wrist. Repeat as necessary.

Find relaxing relief: Press the solar plexus button in the center-point of each hand. (See Chart B, page 11.) With your left hand, wrap your fingers over the top of your right hand, and place the left thumb in the center-point of your right palm. (See Photo 30 on page 185.) Use a slow press-and-release motion to calm the network of nerves throughout your system. Pressing this reflex point will help relax the whole body, ultimately easing pain from the wrist. Repeat on the other hand.

To increase flowing circulation: Give a gentle reflex workout around the entire wrist area. Use the press-and-rotate movement to stimulate a renewed flow of lubricating fluids through the tunnel. Take in a few deep breaths to relax tension throughout the body, and also to oxygenate your blood for faster healing.

To control pain: Notice the reflex point marked "carpal tunnel" in Illustration 16. Press this reflex button from the front and back simultaneously. Hold pressure on this point of the flexion crease for seven seconds and then release for seven seconds. This will help release pain as it flushes out fluid accumulations that have been crowding up into the tunnel. Repeat several times to ease pain.

If your forearm is hurting, use reflex pressure at various stops all the way up your arm. This press-and-rotate method will feel sore, so work slowly and easily, up and down zones two and three of your forearm. (See Chart E on page 14.) This is an easy technique; just apply pressure with your thumb along the invisible zone lines. Press-and-rotate your thumb on each spot for seven seconds, move a half inch up the arm, and work another reflex point for seven seconds, continuing up and around on the shoulder. Repeat on the other arm to balance energy flow.

Continue to Care for Your Hands after Work Hours

Once you have checked out of your workplace for the day, you need to give special care to your hands. Slowly stretch and bend your wrists, fingers, and thumbs every few hours to keep the circulation moving. Massage around each finger and thumb, around your wrist, and up the arm and shoulder. Have your partner or a friend rub your neck, shoulders, arms, back, and around your shoulder blades. This will encourage renewed circulation and help unblock pinched nerves that could be causing numbness or pain in your hands. Next, fold and rub your hands over one another as though you are applying lotion to them.

When your wrist hurts, the pain often gets worse at night, which will interfere with a good night's sleep, and you don't want that. So, make sure your wrists are straight and not bent as you sleep, because this can cut off circulation. You may want to wear a loose wrist splint to hold your hand aligned, but be careful not to wrap it tightly, or the flow of circulation will weaken.

Hand Exercises to Help Eliminate Pain

Elevation of hand: For added stimulation, raise your hands up above your heart. You can rest your elbow on a desk or table in front of you to do this exercise if you are sitting. Raise hands over your head if you are standing. Open your fingers wide, then close them, one finger at a time. Starting with your little finger, close fingers in to make a fist. Now slowly reopen your hand, one finger at a time. Repeat twice or as needed. Shake each hand vigorously to get the circulation moving. This helps relieve tensions, not only in your wrists, but also in your fingers, arms, and shoulders.

Rotate both hands at the wrist. Make circles to the left and then to the right to improve blood flow and drain built-up fluids from your wrist. If you feel a burning pain from your wrists into the middle fingers, or if you are awakened at night because your hands have fallen asleep, elevate them and do the above techniques to eliminate pain.

Backward wrist stretch: Reduce swelling and irritation in tendons by placing your hands together with elbows out. (See Illustration 17.) Press all fingers together and stretch each wrist backward. Gently use your left hand to push back your right wrist, release, and repeat seven times. Then alternate hand pressure, and gently use your right hand to push back the left wrist, release, and repeat seven times.

Most often when using your hands, the fingers are in a forward position, bending toward the inside wrist to do their work, which tightens the wrist nerves. The Backward Wrist Stretch helps bend the wrists and fingers in a reverse position to stretch open the channels for better circulation.

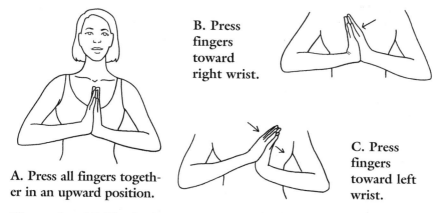

B. Press fingers toward right wrist.

A. Press all fingers together in an upward position.

C. Press fingers toward left wrist.

Illustration 17: The Backward Wrist Stretch will give your wrists relief by reversing their position. It opens energy channels for the tiny electric impulses to travel through the median nerve in the wrist, and encourages better circulation for fast healing. *Tip:* Press base of palms together to rebuild muscle and ligament strength in wrists.

Research Shows Vitamin B$_6$ Helps Relieve CTS

Several medical doctors have done research on the vitamins needed to help prevent carpal tunnel surgeries. They are enthusiastic about the use of Vitamin B$_6$ to cure CTS. John M. Ellis, M.D., a Texas surgeon and family practitioner, and author of five published studies on the deficiency of Vitamin B$_6$, tells of positive results.

He has prescribed high doses of B$_6$ daily to hundreds of patients over the last thirty years, with no negative side effects. When using from 50 to 200 milligrams of Vitamin B$_6$ for at least ninety days, it helped relieve CTS in most cases. However, when the Vitamin B$_6$ supplements were no longer taken, the patients' symptoms returned.

You may want to add natural foods to your diet that are rich in Vitamin B$_6$, such as brewer's yeast, bran cereals, brown rice, whole wheat, tuna, beans, oats, and bananas, to name a few. However, a multiple vitamin supplement may offer you the higher dose needed to stop carpal tunnel problems. Check with your doctor before taking large amounts of Vitamin B$_6$, or any other supplemental vitamin. It could, in some cases, cause a negative reaction or interfere with other medications.

Health tip: Soaking your swollen wrist and hand in cold water will help reduce inflammation. Fill a large storage container, the sink, or tub with cool water and add some crushed ice. Submerge hand and wrist (forearm and elbow if you want) for a few seconds, take out, and repeat several times to encourage normal energy flow and help eliminate swelling and pain.

Tarsal Tunnel Syndrome (TTS) Is Similar to CTS

My grandson loves to run. He is on the track team at school and looks forward to every event with great enthusiasm. The only trouble is that sometimes he develops pain on the inside of his ankle bone and occasionally feels tingling sensations in the soles of his feet. This happens if he forgets and allows his ankles to turn inward while running. This happens because fibrous tissues swell, and the tiny electric impulses that travel the nerve cannot pass through the tarsal tunnel. TTS is similar to CTS, only the pain is in the ankles rather than the wrists.

If you have these symptoms, let me pass this advice to you. Avoid standing, walking, or running with your ankles turned inward, for the nerve energy may not be able to pass and it could cause TTS. Use reflexology to stimulate the electric impulses through the nerves, and elevate your feet when you can. Place Maseur Innersoles in the shoes to enhance blood circulation, and concentrate on walking with your ankles straight.

Body Reflexology Gives Complete Relief from Leg Pain

Dear Mrs. Carter,

I had never tried reflexology until three weeks ago. I had such excruciating pain in my right knee I could barely walk. I have no idea what caused it. I use a quad cane because of polio problems, but had to resort to using two canes to be able to move at all. I had used "over-the-counter drugs," cold and heat to no avail. Could not sleep, was crying with pain. Finally, after a week of this I called my friend in Nevada and asked her to look in her reflexology book (written by you) for help. As she read it to me over the telephone, I applied pressure and thought there was "some" relief.

Mrs. Carter, by the next morning there was *no pain!* And, there has been no pain ever since. It is like a miracle! Two days later I bought your book and have been greedily devouring it! I want to read it through, taking notes and highlighting. Then I intend to start a daily regimen and diet for myself. Thank you for all the time, study, work, and effort you have put into helping others.

Yours truly,

E. H., Texas

CHAPTER 20

How Reflexology Can Help Your Back

The importance of the spine to our general health is familiar to all practitioners. The chiropractic, naturopathic, and osteopathic doctors know that the greater part of one's well-being depends on the condition of the spine.

To work the reflexes of the back, or spine, is to relax the muscle tension surrounding any vertebra that is not in perfect and healthful alignment. Remember that the body can never be in perfect health if the spine is out of alignment.

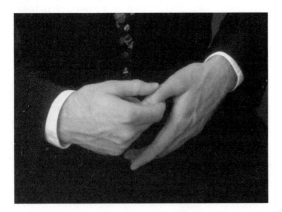

Photo 23: Position for working the cervical spine (neck) reflex area on the left hand.

You reviewed the position of the reflexes in the hands, when you studied Chart B (page 11). Notice in Photo 23 how the thumb of the right hand is working along the edge of the left thumb. This is where the upper spinal reflexes are found in each hand.

There are other reflex points that are equally important when helping heal a sore back. They are the supporting muscles to the spine, and can be found along zones two and three on each hand.

Your spine is not in just one long column, but is divided into 24 dynamic segments that will let you bend over and pick a ball up off the ground. Alternatively, your spine allows you to turn your body from side to side, helping you to get in and out of your car, or to play golf, baseball, tennis, or do other activities that you enjoy.

In between each segment, or disc, are little shock absorbers that cushion the spine when you jump and keep the spinal bones from rubbing together. These discs and the shock absorber fluids can degenerate with age, but you can keep this from happening by using good health habits. Exercise to stay flexible, eat nutritious foods, and use reflexology to encourage healing circulation.

Another way is to avoid lifting heavy items. A general rule is not to lift over thirty pounds after the age of forty. If you have heavy chores, get help from a neighbor, friend, or a family member, or hire someone to do the chores for you, because you do not want to hurt your back. Once it is out of alignment, it may take a long time to straighten out and mend.

HOW TO WORK THE SPINAL REFLEXES

Just as the spinal reflex in the foot follows in one straight line from the big toe down, you will look to the thumb for the spinal reflex and follow down the hand. Notice that the thumb bone represents the spine. It is in a straight line, from just above the first joint in your thumb to the base of thumb, and ending just below the wrist. You will search for tender spots along this area when working reflexes to help the neck and spine.

Remember both thumbs correspond to the spine, which are in zone one. In zones one, two, and three are reflexes to the spinal cord, nerves, and some of the spinal muscles, that keep the back straight. The index and middle fingers correspond to muscles that hold the spine upward and in an erect position.

The cervical spine (neck):   The upper part of the thumb and fingers represent the head and neck of your body. For the upper neck reflex, concentrate on both thumbs from just below the thumbnail to the middle of the two thumb joints. (See Photo 23 on page 142.)

The thoracic spine (upper to mid back):   If there is pain or tension in the upper part of the back, as in your neck or between the shoulders, look for tenderness around the second thumb joint. If you have backaches in the center of your back, then look for tenderness along the center of this reflex area, as in Photo 53, page 281.

Lumbar spine (low back):   If you have lower back trouble, then look for tenderness in the reflex area from the waistline of the hand to the wrist. Work along this area of the thumb with a press-and-rotate motion. When you find a sore spot, work it for a few seconds and then exert pressure all around the area with a press-and-pull technique to relax the surrounding nerves and muscles. Also work along the outside of each hand to benefit hip and pelvis. Extend your reflex work to both hands.

Sacrum and tailbone/coccyx (lower back):   If you suffer from a sore tailbone, you will want to send healing energy to this area of your spine. The reflex that corresponds to the tailbone area is on each wrist. Press and work the whole area of the lower lumbar reflexes (see Photo 24 for lumbar and coccyx) using your thumb and fingers, working all the way around the wrist including the front, back, and sides of both wrists. Notice when you are pressing on the lower lumbar reflex that you are very close to the bladder reflex (see Chart B on page 11).

Spinal muscles: It is equally important to work the reflex area of the back *muscles,* because they pull the body upright into a straight position, and help the spine bend forward and sideways at the waist. Work the reflex areas along all zones to stimulate healing energy to the posterior muscles, rhomboideus, major, and even the trapezius shoulder muscles. All the muscles are interrelated, and work together to keep your spine strong and flexible. See Photo 25, page 145.

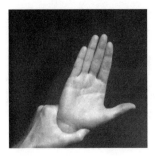

Photo 24: Position for working the reflex to the lower back (coccyx). Apply pressure to the front of wrist and then to the back side of wrist. Work both hands.

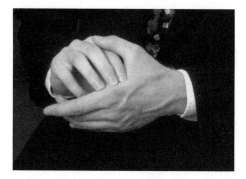

Photo 25: Position for working reflexes that correspond to the back's supporting muscles. Using two or three fingers, apply pressure along zone two and over the back of each hand.

KEY REFLEX AREAS TO HELP HEAL BACK TROUBLES

Using the pressing, rolling motion, or the thumb-walk technique, work your way up and down the ridge of thumb and index finger. Search out the tender spots with your fingers and work them a few seconds. If the problem is in the upper back, neck, or shoulder, work the upper part of both hands. If the problem is in the lower back, work the reflexes in the lower part of each hand that corresponds to the lumbar spine, sciatic nerve, and hip.

Work up and down the index finger which corresponds to the muscles tightly intermingling with the spine. Using the thumb and index finger of the opposite hand, squeeze over the whole area again with a pinching technique to relax all the supporting muscles around the spine.

Work the liver, kidney, and bladder reflex areas on both hands if they are not functioning well; these organs can cause back pain.

In some tender places, you may find it more beneficial just to hold with a steady pressure for a few seconds, especially in the reflexes to the spine. You will soon learn what seems to be the best for your particular case.

With Reflexology, I Was Able to Help My Wife and a Good Friend

Dear Mrs. Carter,

Your book has changed my life. Let me tell you about some of the people I have helped with reflexology. About fifteen years ago, my wife fell from a windowsill while cleaning the windowpane and broke her coccyx. I took her to the doctor and he told us the only way was to operate. I asked him what the chances were concerning the operation . . . he told us 50% recovery. My wife was so frightened, we decided against the operation. However, the damage scarred the bone and caused sagging of the vertebrae, so the spinal cord did not have good support.

My wife started developing bad blood circulation and bad temper, and she did not sleep well. She asked me if there was any way to help her with reflexology. So I decided to really work hard to help her, and I did. That was several years ago, and today she is in perfect health, thanks to you. I love you, Mrs. Carter, and a million thanks from my devoted wife!

Another time I was able to help a dear friend of mine, Doctor H., who had a heart attack and was in a very bad state. I was called and treated him for an hour and what do you know, he was out of danger. I treated him seven more times with reflexology; this was a year ago. And no more heart attack for him, thanks to you.

God bless you and sincerely,

C. L. B., Secunda

Injured Back Helped by Reflexology

Mr. M. reports:

"I received your book on reflexology and have brought about an amazing improvement in my health by using the methods put forth by Mrs. Carter.

"I injured my back several years ago and after using these methods, I have been free of pain for the first time in years. I sleep like a baby and feel years younger. I have treated some of my friends, bringing relief from sinus congestion, sore throats, muscular pains, and so forth.

"I can't thank Mrs. Carter and the publisher enough for putting these wonderful health secrets in print."

COMMON CAUSES OF BACK PAIN

A few years ago, all back trouble was called *lumbago*. We know now that there are many causes of back pain. Besides the vertebra being out of alignment (a slipped or ruptured disc), backache can be caused by malfunctioning kidneys, lack of calcium, female disorders, arthritis, lifestyle changes, muscle spasms, emotional stress, injuries, obesity, osteoporosis, or overexertion. There are also some very serious conditions, such as spina bifida (separated spine), spondylolisthesis (vertebra displacement), scoliosis (curvature of the spine), and accidental occurrences.

Working the reflexes to the spine will help increase circulation to the painful area, and helps relax the posterior muscles surrounding the spinal area. If one side of the back is in pain, work the hand on the same side. You can also work on the webbing between the thumb and index finger as explained in Chapter 4.

Dr. Bowers claims that zone therapy (reflexology) is one of the most valuable methods for treating obstinate conditions. He states, "Lumbago, as a rule, responds very quickly to zone therapy. Cases who come to the office 'all doubled up' are straightened out, frequently in one treatment, and wend their way homeward rejoicing."

Deluxe Hand & Foot Roller helps ease back pain: Another successful method of treating back troubles is the use of the Deluxe Hand & Foot Roller. (See Photo 12C, page 49.) The little roller-fingers will press firmly into the reflexes in the palms. Turn your hands outward, and the pressure will be along zone one.

If your arms get tired of holding the roller, here is a helpful tip: Rest comfortably, and place the roller on a lap tray. Put one hand at a time over the deluxe-roller fingers, and roll it back and forth for a good reflex workout. Refer to Photo 43, on page 254. (You can also place the deluxe roller under each foot, and roll it back and forth along the instep, from the big toe to the heel.) For best results, use the roller on your feet for about fifteen to twenty minutes.

In private practice, I had wonderful results simply by working the reflexes in the feet. Dr. Bowers cites some very amazing results to relieve back pain, also by the use of the reflex comb and clamps, as explained in Chapter 5.

How Reflexology Relieves Minister of Back Pains

A minister who for weeks had been unable to turn in bed without assistance was, after a twenty-minute treatment, able to arise and walk unaided. He was entirely relieved of pain and discomfort within a few hours, and the next day he was "up and around."

Relief almost always follows the first treatment, apparently regardless of the cause of the back trouble.

Man Cured of Back Pain in a Few Minutes

Dr. Bowers tells of a case of backache that had persisted for more than three months. This gentleman had taken practically every form of treatment that could be recommended by the most able specialists; he had even been to Hot Springs. He was bent almost double, and for many weeks had not been able to stand erect. He was given two metal combs and told to squeeze them for ten or fifteen minutes while waiting in the foyer. After he was brought into the office, his hands were thoroughly "combed" by pressure, from finger-tip to wrist. He straightened out completely after his first reflex treatment, and expressed himself as entirely relieved from pain. He received a similar reflexology treatment the following day, after which he went his way rejoicing.

"These results are practically uniform. I know of many patients thus cured with reflexology and a comb," states Dr. Bowers.

Train Conductor Relieved of Back Pain

One doctor, a reflexology enthusiast, while on a trip to a Shriners' convention, noticed that the conductor of the train walked "all doubled up" and seemed to be suffering great pain. It developed that the railroad man had a "misery in his back," had given up work, and gone to an infirmary for three weeks—without obtaining much relief. Three days prior to his resuming work he had not been able to straighten up or make any sudden move without suffering excruciatingly.

He was invited to come to the smoking compartment for a few minutes, where the doctor put strong pressure on the thumb and forefingers of both the trainman's hands. The conductor was not informed of the purpose of this procedure, so his imagination had nothing to work on.

After holding his fingers in this manner for about ten minutes, the whistle blew and the conductor had to leave his chair suddenly. He straightened up and went out on the run. When he came back he laughed and said, "This is the first time in six weeks I've gotten up or moved without pain. What in thunder did that firm pressure have to do with lumbago, anyway?"

The doctor saw the man before leaving the train two hours later, and he was still free from pain.

These results can be duplicated by anyone who will apply the simple techniques outlined in this book.

There are so many natural methods to alleviate suffering and disease that I could go on forever telling you of them.

Reflexology Saves Man from Operation on Spine

One case I had was a man in his thirties, with a back so bad that he was unable to do any manual labor of any kind. I have been in his home when he turned to say "good-bye," and went crashing to the floor. He had to crawl to a chair to help himself slowly up. The doctors told him he had a slipped disc and would only get worse, as the disc was deteriorating and could not possibly get better. They claimed an operation was imperative. I talked him into letting me give him some reflex treatments to see what reflexology could do for him. In a very short time, Mr. B. was free from all back trouble. He was able to do all kinds of manual work, such as roofing his house, hiking, etc. That was seventeen years ago and he still has a good strong back. I wonder how he would be if he had undergone an operation?

CHAPTER 21

How Reflexology Can Help Your Digestive System

Do you remember that huge meal you ate last night? Well, your digestive system had to break it all down, and down, into tiny liquid particles so that it could actually be absorbed into your bloodstream, and then into your cells. This is how body tissues receive their nutrition. Each organ in this grand system has its individual job to do, separating usable nutrients from unusable waste.

The miraculous digestive system includes teeth, mouth, esophagus, stomach, liver, gall bladder, pancreas, large and small intestines, appendix, rectum, and anus. The awesome complexity of this system usually functions twenty-four hours a day with notable efficiency. It requires very little conscious work on our part. All we have to do is gratify our hunger with a pleasant tasting meal, and nature does the rest for us.

Of course, with any large system such as this, things can go wrong. This is the reason we need to pay special attention to what we eat, and use reflexology stimulation to keep this fantastic complex running smoothly. Since we cover most organs of this system in separate chapters, we will refer mostly to the stomach and intestines here.

THE IMPORTANCE OF YOUR STOMACH

Everyone knows what it is to have a stomachache. The stomach is the most abused part of your whole body. It has to take care of everything that is pushed into it through the mouth, and very few people care what they feed into this loyal hard-working servant, or how they present it. Yet after food is received, the stomach strives to accept it, separating and disposing of each separate parcel into the right channel. Just think of all the unhealthy, indigestible liquids containing alcohol, sugar, fats, harmful additives, and acids that also have to be distributed into their proper disposal channels.

Food that goes into the mouth should be chewed well and mixed with saliva, as this is the first stage of digestion. Do you take time to chew your food into a smooth liquid paste before you swallow it? If you do, you probably are enjoying perfect health today and have no need for trying to find a way back to health.

The entry of food into the stomach—as well as its exit—is regulated by circular muscles that alternately expand and contract. The stomach works on the food both mechanically and chemically. The movement of the stomach mashes the food, kneading it as a cook kneads dough. This permits the thorough mixing in of digestive juices, the main ones being pepsin and hydrochloric acid.

You will see in Chart H (on page 164) how the stomach and its related organs work. This will give you some idea of what goes on in various parts of the alimentary canal. With the help of this diagram, you can follow the long journey that food makes through the food canal of your body.

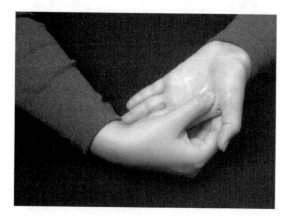

Photo 26: Position for working the stomach reflex area, on the left hand. Press-and-rotate fingers and thumb simultaneously on both sides of hand. Work toward wrist, then across hand.

REFLEX TECHNIQUES TO RELIEVE STOMACH TROUBLES

Since the stomach is located more to the left side, let us start with the reflexes on the left hand. If you will look at Photo 26, you will see how the thumb of the right hand is pressing into the soft spongy area of the left hand, near the lower pad of the thumb and near the webbing. You will work this area with a rolling-pressing motion. If you start to feel nauseated, stop for a few minutes. Take up the right hand and work the same reflex area on it.

Although the stomach lies mostly on the left side of the body, we want to work the same reflexes in both hands. This is because the duodenum, liver, and pancreas extend over to the right side of the body, and their reflexes will be found in the right hand. These organs are all interrelated and depend on each other, and each needs equal reflex attention.

Now let us work the Magical V, which is in the webbing between your thumb and index finger. This special reflex area seems to have a very intimate connection with the stomach. Work close to the thumb, and around the thumb, to stimulate the salivary glands. These glands send saliva into the mouth to moisten your food, thus making it easier to swallow. Saliva actually helps you taste dry foods.

Give a complete reflex workout for the whole body when alleviating stomach troubles. Cover all the reflexes, but focus your attention on any sore spots. If you are working on your own stomach reflex, it may be easier for you to use the knuckle of your right index finger (see Photo 27b, page 172), or a reflexology tool such as the Reflex Probe. Remember, you may start feeling digestive movement in your stomach during the reflex workout, and this is okay, as various responses will occur, depending on your current health condition.

Often when I start working the stomach reflex area on patients, they become uneasy as their stomach starts to gurgle. I just assure them this is a natural reaction. It doesn't hurt, and it proves that the reflex stimulation is causing movement within the abdomen. It has energized the internal action of digestion in breaking down food that the body needs to keep us alive.

After reflex work, many individuals have to use the bathroom immediately following the session; this, too, is a normal, healthy reaction.

The stomach is the central point for the nerves and should be given consideration in all cases of nervousness and nervous exhaustion. Apply firm pressure in the stomach, and solar plexus reflex zones, on the palm of each hand. (See Photo 45, page 261.) The Magic Reflexer can be used here with both hands simultaneously. Place your reflexer between both hands. Position it so that one of its "little fingers" is in the solar plexus reflex point in each hand. (See the star in center of each hand on Chart B, page 11, and refer to Photo 10b, page 42.)

Now that you know the importance your stomach plays in your well being, you will want to find the reflex method that seems to work best for you. Search for tender spots in these areas, and when you find then, *work them out.*

REFLEXOLOGY HELPS RELIEVE MANY DIGESTIVE COMPLAINTS

Reflexology is valuable for those who suffer indigestion, nausea, vomiting, and all forms of stomach disorders. It has also been used successfully in cases of gastric ulcers. Working reflexes to the stomach, as well as working the reflexes described for motion sickness, often helps stop morning sickness caused from pregnancy. (See caution, page 222.)

Heartburn can be relieved by working reflexes to the digestive system. Concentrate on working the stomach, duodenum, and pancreas reflexes in both hands to ease the burning sensation. Work the liver and gall bladder reflex on the right hand to prevent future problems.

Helpful tips to alleviate heartburn: Drink water with raw apple cider vinegar (or fresh lemon juice) in it to ease digestion and assist with detoxification. Learn to eat slowly and in a relaxed environment, never eat when you are emotionally upset, and do not eat too much fatty or spicy foods.

Hernia and indigestion: Both cause a burning sensation, which can be felt behind the breastbone, near the heart. Indigestion causes gas, belching, abdominal cramps, bloating, and heartburn. Both dilemmas can be provoked by tension and stress, and are frequently brought on by fatty or rich foods, too much coffee, chocolate, alcohol, garlic, onions, or smoking.

Many people ask, "What is a hiatus hernia, and what causes it?" We learned in Chapter 11 about our diaphragm; this is a breathing-muscle that divides the upper respiratory system from the lower abdomen. It pushes air out of our lungs. Through the center of this long horizontal muscle is an opening that allows the esophagus to pass through to the stomach.

It is referred to as the "hiatus opening." When the top of the stomach expands, sometimes it inflates up into the hiatus, disturbing the sphincter muscle at the opening of the stomach, and causes it to remain open a bit. This allows excessive gastric acid from the stomach to rise into the esophagus. A burning sensation can be felt near the heart, and occasionally in the left arm, much like the symptoms of a heart attack.

Work across the diaphragm reflex in the center of each hand. Also activate the Magical V reflex section between your thumb and index finger (see Photo 7, page 33, and Photo 58, page 283) to promote healing energy into your abdomen. You may also hold steady pressure here to ease pain.

Use body reflexology: Place your fingertips directly over the diaphragm and solar plexus reflex just below your breastbone to relax its distress. (Use same directions as for hiccups, on page 156.) This is a very important reflex and may be exquisitely tender. Work gently at first, then with a deep rotary pressure here to relax the nerves and nature will do the rest.

Allow gravity to help.   A hiatus hernia will often cause more pain when the body is in a horizontal position. Stand or sit up straight and tilt your head and shoulders backward to open the chest area, giving more room for the hiatus to expand. This will allow the acid to drain with gravity back into the stomach. It may also be a comfort to do some deep breathing exercises, which will keep the diaphragm moving smoothly.

Medical Doctor Stops Stomach Pain in Five Minutes

Charles R. Clapp, M.D., Los Angeles, tells us of Mrs. R., aged 25, who had pain in the epigastric region for three days, using several remedies without any relief. "I treated the thumb and index finger of the right hand with no result. When I began on the thumb of the left hand, she said with a smile, 'There, that strikes the spot.' In less than five minutes, she was free from pain and has had no return of same. This is another clincher for attacking the correct zone (reflex)."

Doctors Tell of Ulcer Cures with Reflexology

Dr. Reid Kellogg has cured several cases of ulcers in one to ten treatments, and many others in two or three months, such as those with dangerous hemorrhages and other distressing symptoms. Dr. Kellogg used pressures on the thumb, first, and second fingers of both hands.

Dr. Bowers tells us, "In less than a dozen treatments, many patients were able to retain food, and practically conduct the entire subsequent course of their own cure." He further states, "I want to emphasize that these cases were most grave, and that they had received skilled medical attention for many weeks without apparent benefit."

Reflexology Put Harmony Back Into Life

Dear Mildred Carter,

To make this short is difficult because there is so much to thank you for. With your guidance, I put harmony back into my body through your books. I have read and studied all your books for over two years now. You are my mentor.

I am proud and very happy to practice reflexology from your teachings. It works! I appreciate your personal advice on chewing. It took me several weeks and a lot of practice, and I am just fine now, but a strange thing happened. I started eating sauerkraut as suggested in your book and no longer wanted to smoke. Four weeks have passed and I feel like I never smoked before, and do not feel I ever want to start again. I feel reflexology has made my life simple, healthy, and happy. Thanks for putting my life in harmony. Your books are wonderful. I am forever grateful.

Sincerely,

Joan E.

Reflex Help for Hiccups

Many devious ways have been used to end the annoyance of hiccups, which in some cases has become quite serious, even sending the victim to the hospital.

We will work the webbing in the Magical V and down into the stomach. Then work across the diaphragm reflex areas on both hands. If you still have no relief, use the tongue-pulling method by simply sticking out your tongue as far as possible and holding it there. In this way, you can cure the spasmodic contraction of the diaphragm (the cause of hiccups) by influencing the zone in which the trouble originated.

The best way to get rid of hiccups is with body reflexology. It is easy and always works quickly. Last summer, for instance, we were camping with several families when my daughter-in-law got a very bad case of hiccups. The burps were becoming so severe that they were hurting her ribs and throat. I told her to press her three middle fingers into her stomach, just over the diaphragm (between the sternum "breastbone" and navel), hold for a few seconds, and at the same time, take in a deep breath. That was all it took; her hiccups were gone in one minute.

How Reflexology Helps Stop Motion Sickness

Air, car, and sea can cause a terrible upset stomach and motion sickness. This can definitely ruin the fun. Nevertheless, it can be overcome with the help of reflexology. We learn that it is caused mainly from a gland in the inner ear. By looking at the Zone Chart on page 14, you will see that zones three, four, and five run through the inner and outer ear canals. So working on the third, fourth, and fifth fingers will stimulate this area.

Another reflex to help stop motion sickness and relieve nausea is in the arm. This button is approximately one-and-a-half inches from the wrist, in the center of your forearm. Hold firm pressure until all signs of illness are gone.

I suggest you experiment a little here and find the method that best suits your specific condition. Give each method a chance for ten minutes before going on to another. Remember that the Magical V is an all-important reflex to the stomach.

I do not recommend the Magic Reflexer in motion sickness cases, as it stimulates all the internal organs. In this case, we want to soothe the stomach, not stimulate it. Steady pressure with the reflex comb or the clamps can be used for this purpose. I have even held the ends of my fingers between my teeth when there was nothing better to hold pressure on several fingers at a time.

How Reflexology Saved Travelers from Car Sickness

A friend from the East Coast flew out West with her father for a visit with us. We planned to show them the beautiful scenery of Oregon, and decided to travel along the coast by car. Sue was afraid to go, as she knew the roads were winding and snakelike. I asked her if she would mind trying reflexology. She agreed to take a chance and put reflex therapy to the test, as she loves the ocean and very much wanted to see the Pacific.

We experimented and found that by rubbing the middle, ring, and little fingers (in the ear reflex zone) all signs of carsickness ceased. Sue was able to travel every place from that day on without the fear of being sick. We took her and her father several hundred miles over the next few days; they had a wonderful time sightseeing and took dozens of pictures. No one got sick; we all had a lot of fun, and have many great memories.

How to stop baby's crying with reflexology: These methods may be used anytime the baby is crying. Use a gentle pressure on the stomach and Magical V reflexes; press on the back and palm of each hand, using your thumb and index fingers. Another way to calm baby is to very softly stroke over their little hands and arms with your fingertips, and then with the flat side of your fingernails. If their shoes are off, a gentle pressure to the top and sole of their tiny feet works wonders.

THE SIGNIFICANCE OF THE LARGE AND SMALL INTESTINES

The biggest part of your digestive system is the large and small intestines. The small intestine is actually long and narrow; it measures approximately 18 to 23 feet long, depending on the individual. The larger intestine (or colon) is much wider, but is only about 5 to 6 feet long. They are all coiled up to fit inside a small space in the abdomen, similar to how a long rope fits into a small basket.

Taking care of bowel troubles: You know the importance of keeping the outside of your body clean; it is just as important to keep your inside systems clean, too. A regular cleansing of the intestines is a requirement for good health. It is especially important to remove toxins and hazardous bacteria. These offenders prevent the body from absorbing nutrients from the digestive tract. When the bacterial balance in the intestine is upset, it can cause diarrhea. This is the body's natural attempt to get rid of irritating or poisonous matter.

How to find the reflexes to the intestines: Some students become overwhelmed when they learn about all the different names that are attached to the intestines. Look at Chart A (page 10) for a moment and you will see there are small and large intestines, ascending, transverse, descending, and sigmoid colons. This does sound like a lot to learn. However, when looking at Chart B (page 11), you will see reflexes that correspond to this area are all within the heel pad of each palm. Therefore, when you do hand reflexology, it will be easy. Just work across these pads to stimulate healing energy to all parts of your intestines. (See Illustration 18, below, and Photo 69, page 288.)

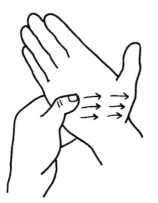 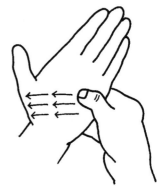

Working the Right Hand   Working the Left Hand

Illustration 18: Work the reflex area across the lower part of right and left hands to activate healing energy to the corresponding large and small intestines.

REFLEXOLOGY HELPS STIMULATE BETTER INTESTINAL HEALTH

A total reflex workout helps promote digestive juices, which are needed to move bulk and waste. Concentrate on working across the middle and lower sections of both palms to stimulate internal healing energy from your waistline down to the rectum. This will stimulate both small and large intestines. Also, work up and down the spinal reflex on each hand several times.

The Magic Reflexer or the Deluxe Hand & Foot Roller can be an advantage here in helping you stimulate these reflexes, as their "little fingers" can do all the work for you. By using reflexology and eating the right foods, you will not need to resort to harmful laxatives for alleviating the discomforts of a troubled colon.

Diarrhea: If you have recently suffered from diarrhea, increase your fluid intake to replace lost liquids, and do not eat fatty foods that will irritate the colon. Enzymes from fresh fruits and vegetables are essential to proper digestion and good health.

Constipation: If you suffer with constipation, you need to eat more fiber and more raw foods. This will help add the enzymes that your body needs to break up bulk and fats from your meal. Eat less sugar, flour, rice, and pasta as they can cause a sluggish intestine.

Years ago I learned something from Dr. Marsh Morrison that I often share with my patients, and now I will share it with you. Back in the old days, people just had to squat behind trees or bushes when it was time to empty their colon. It was a rough life, but actually, putting the body in this position made it easy for them to quickly evacuate the bowels.

With only the front part of their feet and toes touching the ground, the sigmoid colon and rectum straightened a little from its bent contour into a more suitable position for bowel movements. Now I am sure you do not want to squat in the woods. However, remember this the next time you go to the bathroom. After you sit down, raise your heels off the floor, and bring your knees up, so that you feel your bowels elongate. You may be pleasantly surprised at how quickly waste matter is excreted.

Reflexology Has Been Stopping Pain for Many Years

A report was given by Orin W. Joslin, M.D., Medical Director of Dodgeville General Hospital and Pine Grove Sanatorium, in Dodgeville, Wisconsin.

January 5, 1918

We have been using zone therapy (reflexology) as a routine measure in our hospital and sanatorium, especially for pain, and we very seldom fail to get satisfactory results. We hardly ever think of using morphine any more. We have never had a case of gas

pains that did not respond inside of ten minutes to zone therapy
(reflexology).

Reflexology Will Continue to Stop Pain for Many Years

A large number of doctors and hospitals use reflexology today. It
is referred to as a complementary therapy to post- and pre-surgery.
Many conscientious doctors are interested in this natural art of healing for their patients. We often hear from doctors who are using
reflexology on themselves, each other, and their families, to learn
what secrets the reflexes can tell them about their health.

A program titled "Healing from the Heart" was recently shown
on ABC's "Good Morning America." M. Oz, M.D., talked of combining complementary medicines of the East and West in his Cardiac
Care Center at a hospital in New York. Dr. Oz will be heading the
program that offers nutrition, acupuncture, massage, energy healing,
reflexology, and prayer at this holistic hospital of the future.

Dr. Clapp says, "I could give many case histories to show why I
am so enthusiastic over zone therapy (reflexology). I never would
have believed what it can do if I had not actually seen and done the
work myself. I am more than delighted with it."

I know how Dr. Clapp felt, because in all the years I was practicing reflexology, I never failed to be astonished at the miracles of
healing it brought forth without anything more than stimulating the
reflexes with the fingers for a few minutes. It seemed like working
magic, but, truly, I was only giving the magic of nature a helping hand
in her efforts to release congested channels so that her healing forces
could revive glandular activity.

CHAPTER 22

A Journey Through the Alimentary Canal

All the food you eat and enjoy takes a specific journey through your fascinating body. It travels through the alimentary canal, a prime source of power that converts and channels nutrients where needed to keep the body functioning. When studying reflexology, it is important to understand how this system operates.

With the help of Chart H (page 164), you can follow the long journey that food takes through the alimentary canal, or food canal, of your own body. You will discover the various stages of your digestive system, and the work that progresses in different parts of the canal. This visual chart and its explanations will be helpful as you use reflexology to bring relief from any malfunction in this area.

EASY-TO-FOLLOW EXPLANATIONS OF THE DIGESTIVE SYSTEM

The first stage of digestion is chewing food into small pieces with your teeth, and allowing it the chance to mix with liquid saliva before you swallow. It takes an average meal approximately 12 to 24 hours to go through various stages of digestion. Of course, liquids travel through the kidneys and bladder within one or more hours. Each person's system is different. Digestive time depends on what type of food was eaten, the person's age and size, how active the person is, and what type of health the person is in.

Salivary glands: First the food is put into your mouth, where it is cut up and ground by the action of the teeth, then pressed against the palate by the tongue. Dry food is moistened and softened by juices secreted by the salivary glands. There are three different types of glands: those under the tongue, those near the jaw, and those near the inner ear; and each produces a different kind of salivary juice. The process of chewing your food will take from 5 to 120 seconds, depending on whether you are eating soft food like pudding, dry crackers, or a hard carrot.

Esophagus: Now in a softened state, the food slides down the ten-inch esophagus into the stomach. This process only takes about twelve seconds.

Stomach: During its stay here, gastric (digestive) juices, produced at the rate of over six pints a day, soften foods further until it reaches the consistency of a paste. From time to time, a valve opens and allows small quantities of this paste to pass into the curving tube of the duodenum. The stomach mixes, mashes, and stirs food for about three and a half to four hours.

Duodenum: The duodenum is the first ten inches that lead from the stomach into the small intestine. Here, bile from the liver and gall bladder, plus pancreatic juices from the pancreas, come through and continue the digestive process into yet smaller particles.

Liver: The liver is the largest organ in the whole body, weighing between three and four pounds, and carries a complicated network of tiny bile canals and blood vessels. It removes waste and destroys harmful poisons, and it sends them away through the kidneys. Every day the liver produces about one and three-quarter pints of bile, most of which collects in the gall bladder before passing through the bile duct into the small intestine. It works closely with the gall bladder, pancreas, and small intestine for five to six hours cleaning food-filled blood, storing sugar, and manufacturing bile that digests fats.

Pancreas: The pancreas produces an alkaline fluid (pancreatic juices) that helps to convert starch, proteins, and fats into chemical compounds used by the body. It also produces insulin, which controls the way the body makes use of sugar.

Small intestine: Soaked with bile and pancreatic juice, the food-paste now passes into the small intestine, which itself produces close to a pint of digestive juices each day. The small intestine contains many small cone-like structures that act as pumps, extracting most of the usable part of the food-paste. It also has many muscles that expand and contract, pushing along the unusable food, much as the squeezing of a tube pushes along toothpaste. Food from the small intestine is processed and broken down into very small particles in about four hours. The bloodstream absorbs the usable parts; the rest becomes waste and is delivered into the large intestine.

Large intestine: Also called the colon, this organ squeezes the unusable food along very slowly, extracting water from it on the way. This process takes five to seventeen hours. An important constituent of the body is water, accounting for between sixty and seventy percent of an adult's weight (less in an overweight person, as fat weighs more than water). The importance of consuming an adequate supply of water daily cannot be overemphasized.

Rectum and anus: Waste is stored in the rectum for several hours, usually about seven to ten. However, in some people it can stay for twenty hours or more, if they are constipated. It is eventually pushed into the anus, where it is expelled from the body.

We Learn a Truth from Studying the Digestive System

The truth is, "You really are what you eat and drink!" We eat food because we get hungry and because it tastes so good. Nevertheless, keep in mind there is more to it than that. Nourishment from food provides us with warmth, energy, and the fuel needed to keep our blood clean, our cells strong, and our body growing.

So let's sustain our bodies with foods that will benefit our health, that we can live and enjoy life to the fullest. In addition, remember that reflex stimulation will bring a vigorous new life force to the organs and glands for a healthy body and a happy soul.

All the foods you eat and enjoy take a specific journey through your fascinating body. Here is an easy-to-follow illustration. You will discover the various stages of how your digestive system works.

Remember, this is only one of the remarkable systems of your body. There are nine others that all work together to make you the special person that you are.

A Visual Chart of the Alimentary Canal

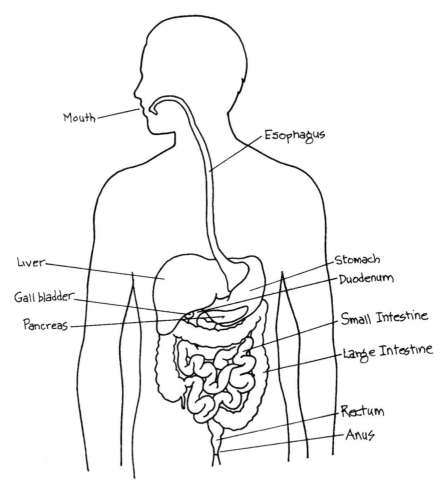

Chart H: We receive our mental and physical nourishment through this important food-carrying system. Refer to this chart as you do reflexology to any of these significant organs.

CHAPTER 23

Reflexology Help for Diabetes and Hypoglycemia

If you are one of the millions who are suffering from diabetes or hypoglycemia, you are aware that malfunctioning of the pancreas is most likely the cause of your disease. The pancreas is one of your endocrine glands, and the majority of its gland cells secrete enzymes needed for digestion.

THE IMPORTANCE OF THE PANCREAS

In the middle of the pancreatic tissue are small islands of different cells that produce a secretion called *insulin*, and this substance flows directly into the bloodstream. It reaches all parts of the body and controls the body's use of sugar. If something goes wrong with the pancreas, these tiny islands quit working properly, the sugar in our blood increases, and we become ill with the disease called *diabetes mellitus*. Scientists have shown that this disease frequently arises because of the lack of minute amounts of the hormone insulin from these vitally important gland cells.

Hypoglycemia is caused by the opposite; when the pancreas is in malfunction, it can also produce too much insulin, thus causing low blood sugar. Doctors are now learning that this is the root cause of several diseases.

HOW TO STIMULATE THE PANCREAS
WITH REFLEXOLOGY

If you will look on Chart G, page 57, you can see how the pancreas extends across the center of the body. It is about six inches long, and wider at one end. The wider end is cradled next to the duodenum. The pancreas lies below the liver and behind the stomach.

If you look at Chart B, page 11, you can see that the pancreas will be stimulated when reflex work is given to the center of one hand (stomach reflex area). Remember that the locations of reflexes in the hands correspond to their mirror image of the organs and glands in the body.

HOW REFLEXOLOGY HELPS
DIABETICS FEEL BETTER

Diabetes is often referred to as *sugar diabetes* because the body has a hard time processing sugars and starches. Insulin is a hormone secreted by the pancreas to help cells use sugar as fuel. When a deficient islet (part of pancreas) does not produce enough insulin, diabetes results.

There are two forms of diabetes: *Diabetes insipidus* is a very rare deficiency of the pituitary hormone that causes a metabolic disorder. The more common form is *diabetes mellitus*, of which there are two types. Type I, or juvenile diabetes, develops in young children and is insulin-dependent. Type II is non–insulin-dependent, and the body is not able to use insulin efficiently. It normally occurs during adulthood. Both can be controlled with medication for most patients. The proper diet is very important to help normalize the systems of the body; exercise is significant as it burns up sugar; and reflexology is excellent, as it increases circulation. Moreover, we know that circulation is vital to providing your cells with oxygen and nutrients, which is essential to their survival.

Tests done at Beijing Medical University in China proved reflexology was an effective treatment for Type II diabetes mellitus. Refer to my book *Healing Yourself with Foot Reflexology* for more information on this study.

If you are afflicted with diabetes, make sure you keep track of your blood sugar level when doing reflex workouts. Many times when using reflexology (especially when the adrenal and pancreas are stimulated), insulin hormone secretions may rise, as the pancreas produces more of the natural insulin hormone.

In some cases, the pancreas *does* produce adequate amounts of insulin, but somehow the body does not absorb it into the cells, and it accumulates in the bloodstream, then is excreted with urine. This is another reason why reflexology is so valuable; it keeps the cells stimulated and the blood moving, which restores harmony and balance to all functions of the body.

Since the adrenal cortex produces steroids, it has to work properly to regulate the blood sugar throughout your body. Did you know that every tissue in your body needs the energy of insulin, except for those in the brain? Therefore, you see how important insulin is to your complete well-being and good health.

Remember: The adrenal and pancreas are just part of the endocrine system, so do not neglect to stimulate the reflexes to all of these hormone-producing glands to help balance the glucose levels. If you can awaken the endocrine glands back into normal function, then you will no longer need the synthetic insulin. However, only your doctor can be the judge of this.

Work reflexes of the digestive system (see Chapter 21) to help release glucose into the bloodstream. Double-check the liver reflex for tenderness; this is where glucose cells are stored until needed for fuel. Remember, the reflex to the liver is located on your right hand. Also, work on the Magical V, the webbing between your thumb and index finger. (See Photo 58.)

In addition, work all the reflexes to the urinary system. The kidneys filter glucose from blood, and the bladder releases excess sugar through the urine, and out of the body, which is most important to your health.

Press-and-release the solar plexus reflex in the center of each hand to relax nerves. (See Photo 45, page 261.) Relaxation will help regulate your blood sugar level. Reflexology helps nature in her attempt to heal the body by reactivating the vital life force back into these congested areas. It is safe and easy to use, even for children.

Give a complete reflex workout and re-check your eye reflexes in each hand for soreness, because diabetic eye disease can result from high blood sugar. In addition, obesity, high blood pressure, heart problems, kidney trouble, or nerve damages could all occur from complications of diabetes. Now you can see why it is so important to use reflexology and take all the steps necessary to control diabetes.

Key health tips for those with diabetes: Do not allow yourself to become overweight, because the heavier you are, the more insulin you may need. Reflexology and regular physical activities play an important role in reducing the risk of further complications by increasing your circulation and helping to keep the blood sugar level closer to normal.

It is critical to stay on your special diet low in sugars and high in greens, onions, garlic, and fibrous roughage to lower blood sugar. Reports from the American Diabetes Association show a daily supplement of 1,000 mg of chromium picolinate activates enzymes, helping to metabolize glucose, moving it from the blood, into cells. It actually lowers blood cholesterol and blood sugar levels in Type II diabetes, and it does not have the yeast base to which so many people are allergic.

I have seen some amazing things happen, which surprised me many times, when the doctor said it could not be done. So, I say, have faith in nature and reflex your way back to health.

Reflexology Used for Thirty-three Years

Dear Mildred Carter:

Reflexology is not new to me, for I have been using it thirty-three years, not professionally, but on myself. It will do all you say it can do.

I'm never sick and never see a doctor, nor do I use drugs of any kind.

Thank you,

L.M.W.

Reflex Cures Condition of Forty Years

Gentlemen:

On March 4th of this year you sent me a copy of Mrs. Carter's book *Healing Yourself with Foot Reflexology.*

I think you should know that it is the best investment I ever made in my life! I will not bore you with the gruesome details, but it effected a cure of a condition, with which I have been troubled for over forty years.

Thankfully,

Mrs. H. M. B., Ohio

Reflexology Brought Relief

Dear Mrs. Carter:

I let my daughter take my book on reflexology. I want another one. I had such good results by using your book on myself. I was nearly crippled with something in my hip and leg, down to my knee. I have spent a lot of money on doctors, and did not get much relief until I got your book on reflexology.

Now I am all right. Thanks to you.

Mrs. A. S. M.

How Reflexology Helps Hypoglycemia Victims

Millions of people are unaware that they are suffering from hypoglycemia (low blood sugar), which may masquerade as a neurosis and many other ailments.

In their book *Low Blood Sugar and You,* Carlton Fredericks, Ph.D., and Herman Goodman, M.D., give us some startling facts of how millions are unaware that they are suffering from some form of hypoglycemia. They claim hypoglycemia is one of man's most dangerous and most unrecognized illnesses, and tell us, "It has gone unidentified as a root cause of both minor and major physical and emotional problems for years."

An unbelievable array of symptoms is caused by low blood sugar. It can turn a balanced person into an apprehensive hypochondriac. It can make a psychiatric wreck out of a normal, well-adjusted individual. It creates intolerable anxiety. The symptoms of low blood sugar not only resemble neurosis or psychosis, they also perfectly imitate epilepsy, migraine headache, peptic ulcer, rheumatoid arthritis, insomnia, asthma, and other allergies. Low blood sugar can cause some of the "side reactions" blamed on drugs. It can directly cause alcoholism, and can possibly lead to drug addiction.

Dr. Goodman and Carlton Fredericks tell us, "Low blood sugar is too infrequently not detected in a complete medical checkup, and when it *is* recognized, the treatment prescribed for it by physicians, forty years behind the times, is the recommendation of more sugar, which is the opposite of what the patient needs, and makes every symptom worse."

We are all aware that glands may be normal, overactive, or underactive. This brings us to the pancreas, which we know to be one of the endocrine glands. If this gland is underactive, it causes diabetes. But few have even given thought to what happens if the pancreas becomes *overactive*. A diabetic is given insulin to keep the blood sugar down to normal levels. We have all heard of the dramatic and disquieting results of taking too much insulin which causes the blood sugar to lower too much and too fast.

So what happens if the pancreas is overactive? It is producing too much insulin and is over-responsive to sugar. Many doctors mistakenly prescribe sugar for the hypoglycemic, which actually puts him in more danger than if he had diabetes. Many unsuspecting sufferers of low blood sugar walk around in insulin shock in a lesser or greater degree, not realizing what the trouble is.

This can be infinitely horrible—all the more so when the sufferer doesn't know what's wrong, can't find out, and winds up diagnosed as a neurotic, hypochondriac, eccentric, "nut," or a chronic invalid. Think of the thousands of poor souls whose lives have been ruined, when they may have only been suffering from a malfunctioning pancreas, and low blood sugar.

Seale Harris, M.D., says, "The low blood sugar of today is the diabetes of tomorrow."

HOW TO WORK THE REFLEXES FOR HYPOGLYCEMIA

Now let us look to reflexology to help us overcome this little understood, but dangerous, disease of our modern day. It doesn't matter if the gland is overactive or underactive. Reflexology is the only medium I know of that will enable the glands to return to their normal state of functioning, aside from proper diet as given in *Low Blood Sugar and You.*

As I have explained in other chapters, the endocrine glands are all interrelated, so if the pancreas is in malfunction, it is out of harmony with the other hormone-producing glands. To help the sufferer of hypoglycemia, we will work the reflexes to the pituitary, pancreas, and adrenal glands, and then all the other endocrine glands as well.

By looking at your Endocrine Chart on page 57, you will see that these reflexes are located in both hands. Using a press-and-rotate technique with your thumb or knuckle will help you find tender reflexes. (See Photo 27.) The pancreas reflex will be very tender if it is not functioning correctly. A good hormonal balance of all glands is important to correct the functioning of the pancreas.

Work reflexes to the digestive system (refer to Chapter 21) to help balance glucose in the bloodstream. Glucose cells are stored in the liver until needed for fuel, so check the liver reflex for tenderness. Remember, it is on the right hand. This will help the body improve digestion and flush out acid wastes. Be sure and work well in this whole area when there are symptoms of hypoglycemia. Also, work on the Magical V section between your thumb and index finger. If you are using the Magic Reflexer, this will give an equal amount of stimulation to all glands, as you roll it around in your hands.

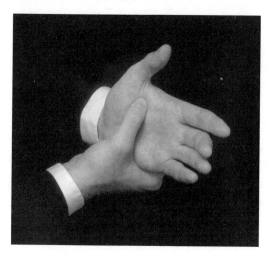

Photo 27a: Position for working the pancreas reflex on the left hand.

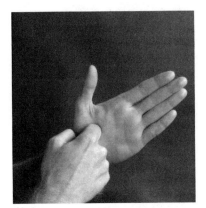

Photo 27b: If fingers are weak or tired, use your knuckle to press-and-rotate on the reflex area. This position gives added strength to the reflex of the pancreas.

Health tips to help those with hypoglycemia: In low blood sugar, the pancreas produces too much insulin and therefore you may become irritable, nervous, depressed, or lethargic. Use reflexology for stress reduction and eat smaller, healthier meals. These are two ways to help correct hypoglycemia.

To control mood swings, it is important to omit sugar, pastries, sodas, and fried foods from your diet. Instead of large meals, try to eat six or seven small meals each day. Eat foods that include high fiber breads and cereals, also fresh vegetables such as broccoli, peas, and garlic. A kiwi fruit or banana, both high in potassium, and natural sugars, blended in a glass of orange juice, is a great combination to quickly bring up low blood sugar fast.

The next time you get a strong craving for sweets, remember that you must love yourself and your family more than you do that piece of cake or bowl of ice cream. If you do eat it, you will probably get a headache or have a negative mood swing. So make the choice: a few minutes of sweets in your mouth will taste good; what about the fact that you may suffer hours afterwards from a painful headache or a grouchy disposition? Then you, and those around you, would be miserable. Is it worth it? The decision is yours.

How a Doctor Recovered after Three Years of Illness

Dr. Stephen Gyland tells of his experience of illness that lasted through three years of suffering.

If all physicians would read the work of Dr. Seale Harris, . . . thousands of persons would not have to go through what I did. I was examined by fourteen specialists and three nationally known clinics before a diagnosis was made by a six-hour glucose (sugar) tolerance test. Previous diagnoses having been brain tumor, diabetes, and cerebral arteriosclerosis. . . . Since then I have used this hard-earned knowledge in diagnosis and curing the condition in numerous patients.

If you or any one you know seems to have an illness that has not been correctly diagnosed, think of hypoglycemia. Don't depend completely on reflexology—demand a six-hour glucose test. Then, with the proper sugar-free diet, let reflexology revitalize the malfunctioning glands back to normal, thus bringing harmony and health back into your whole body.

CHAPTER 24

How to Take Care of Your Appendix and Ileo-cecal Valve

While it is true fewer people are dying from appendicitis, the number of people who suffer from this disease is the same as ever. Acute appendicitis attacks are sudden and give little forewarning. Generally, appendicitis pain will first be noticed around the navel region, then a recurring sharp pain moves to the lower-right section of the abdomen, where the appendix is located.

If there is infection here, it will produce a tight feeling in the muscles and pain between the navel and the right hip. Other symptoms are usually flu-like, such as vomiting, fever, and chills. The *Pfizer Spectrum*, a drug trade magazine, reports that appendectomies are still the most frequently performed operations.

HELP STOP APPENDICITIS WITH REFLEXOLOGY

In using reflexology to the appendix, let us look at Photo 28. See how the left thumb is pressed into the lower side of the right hand. If this spot is tender when you press on it firmly, then it could be an indication of a congested appendix. Work this spot by digging the edge of your thumb in, with a press-and-rotate motion.

If an attack is indicated, and the symptoms do not subside in a few minutes after reflex stimulation is applied, place ice packs over the painful area on the lower right side of the abdomen to ease the pain. Then contact your doctor, or go to the hospital emergency room immediately. If the appendix were to rupture, poisonous bacteria would flow into the system, which can be life threatening.

If this reflex is only slightly tender, you can help reduce the inflammation, and possibly save your appendix from surgery, by working its reflex point on the right hand. Work the reflex area across the lower half of both hands to assure a healthy colon.

Working the reflex to the liver, also on the right hand, will help flush out toxins. You will want to work the reflexes of both kidneys to clear the digestive system, as well as the reflex areas to the thyroid and adrenal glands, to help ward off possible irritability and fatigue.

If the tenderness does not lessen in two or three days, there may be an indication of infection. You should have the attention of your doctor to make sure there is no immediate danger.

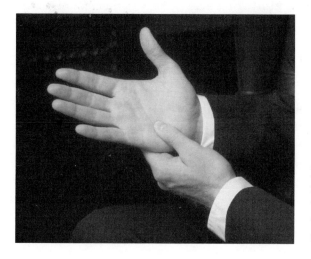

Photo 28: Position for working the reflex to the appendix and the ileo-cecal valve, on the right hand.

To avoid trouble with the appendix: Do not let yourself become constipated. Make time for complete bowel movements when needed. Do not hurry the important event of total elimination. Avoid the use of laxatives, if possible, as they will drain all natural fluids and remove friendly bacteria from your colon. Take them only when necessary. Walking will help encourage bowel movements.

Eat lots of fresh fruits and bran, and drink fluids to give your body natural fiber, enzymes, and Vitamin C. This is a good combination helpful in preventing constipation, fighting off infection, and building up the immune system. Avoid fried foods, as they can get backed up in the intestines.

If there is any type of infection in the body, there may be a problem with bad breath. Use the Stirling Tongue Wand to clean bacteria off your tongue. (See Photo 64, page 286.) Then turn the wand around and use the opposite end to probe your tongue. (See Photo 65, page 286.) Press down and observe whether there is a coating on the tongue. If there is, it could mean poor colon/bowel health, which is not good for the appendix.

Actually, the appendix is kind of like the tonsils. Each one could be removed without your body missing it much. However, if you can keep them it is to your advantage, as they each give strength to your power of immunity.

You will see by looking at your charts that the appendix is located between zones four and five. To help nature further her effort in reviving glandular activity, work on the ring and little finger, and the webbing between these two fingers. Reflex up and down the fourth and fifth zones of your right hand.

Reflex clamps may be used on the fourth and fifth fingers. Also your Magic Reflexer can be of help here. Place the Magic Reflexer in your right hand; place one of its "strong fingers" in the appendix reflex point. Now lace your fingers together with the reflexer between hands and press the heels of both hands together. (See Photo 10b, page 42.) This is a very simple and effective way to hold steady pressure on the appendix and ileo-cecal valve reflex points.

ALLERGIES AND THE ILEO-CECAL VALVE

Because the reflexes to this little valve are located in almost the same place as the appendix, it will be treated with the same reflex technique in the same place. In many cases, tenderness in this area of the right hand, and on the right foot, will indicate that there is inflammation of the ileo-cecal valve instead of the appendix. It will probably take several reflex sessions of working this area to dissipate the inflammation.

How to overcome allergies: This is the button you will press if you are trying to overcome allergies of any kind. It was found that this valve was red and inflamed in every case of allergy when operations were performed on accident victims.

These reflexes can take a lot of massage work without doing any harm; *so if it is sore, rub it out!*

Some Positive Comments from Readers

Dear Mrs. Carter,

Mrs. M. and I feel that you are our friend through your rich sharing with us in the book on foot reflexology.

In the middle thirties we were ministers in Rochester, N.Y. The president of the board was Mr. G. About twenty years later I returned to Rochester for a visit, and while in the home of Mr. and Mrs. G., they told us of a new magic in healing which they had heard about and tested and were made believers, and it was all about a technique of working on the feet.

We forgot about the incident until recently we learned about your book and ordered it. I have been reading and studying it diligently (my wife says she thinks I am reading it more than the Bible).

May God continue to bless you in your continued ministry of healing.

Sincerely and gratefully,

Rev. L.M.

Dear Mrs. Carter:

I have your book *Healing Yourself with Foot Reflexology* and I think it is the best book investment I have ever made. I think it is wonderful and I know it took a lot of your time to compile. God loves you for it!

Thank you and God bless you.

Wilma V., Texas

Dear Ms. Carter,

My sister-in-law got your book on foot reflexology, and she is so happy with it. She never takes sleeping pills any more, and is not gaining much needed weight. No more pain in her legs, and no more pills for elimination. Now I want your book, and I can't wait to receive it!

Ms. S.M.R.

Dear Mildred Carter,

Thank you so very much and may God bless you, Mildred Carter, for your fine work. My group of friends are enjoying much fine health today, because of you.

Sincerely yours,

Mrs. T. T., Canada

To Mrs. M. Carter:

After working on a computer all day, I often come home tired and with a headache. I put the Deluxe Hand & Foot Roller under my feet, and within twenty to thirty minutes, I am completely relaxed and the headache is gone. I appreciate your work. Thank you for the secret of natural healing.

Mr. G. A.

CHAPTER 25

How Reflexology Can Heal Hemorrhoids

I explained in my earlier book, *Healing Yourself with Foot Reflexology,* that reflexes to the rectum are located along the bony edge of the heel and the lower inside edge of the foot. If you have hemorrhoids, you will find a sore spot in this area. When the soreness is worked out, the hemorrhoids will also vanish. When doing hand reflexology, you will locate this reflex on the lower inside edge of the hand, as well as across the bony edge at the wrist.

Since hemorrhoids are swollen veins in the rectum and around the anus, we will look at Chart A, page 10, and the Zone Chart, page 14, to see how meridian zone one goes through the rectum and anus. Therefore, we will work mainly on the reflexes in zone one. As your large colon travels down the left side of the lower abdomen, the last few inches is referred to as the rectum, and waste is expelled from the anus. Therefore, in working the reflex for hemorrhoids, you will work both hands, but especially the left.

Use the press-and-rotate method as you try to feel out tender spots; then change to the other hand for assistance and work it in the same way. You may find that the tenderness is on just one side because the swollen vein is usually on the side, rather than in the center of the rectum/anus area.

Now, take your right thumb and work the inside of your left forearm. Stay in zone one (thumb side of hand) and work from the wrist to about halfway to the elbow to encourage renewed circulation. Use this same method on both forearms.

VICTIMS OF HEMORRHOIDS SUFFER IN SILENCE

Hemorrhoids are one of the most painful conditions and are usually suffered in silence by those who have them. Yet, they are among the quickest ailments to respond to treatments of reflexology.

Hemorrhoids (commonly known as piles) are nothing more than congested veins. There are two types: internal and external. They are the cause of much suffering and inconvenience. At times, they may protrude and cause excessive bleeding. Avoid hemorrhoids by eating more high-fiber foods and drink plenty of fluids to keep your stools soft. Clean yourself with a moist tissue or a damp washcloth, then thoroughly dry yourself afterwards.

For a very painful condition: You can take a sitz bath, or use crushed ice packs on the area. If you take a hot sitz bath, make sure to have cool water on the side to dip your hands into and apply to your face, head, over the shoulders, or back. This will help keep you from getting too hot or dizzy.

For anal itching: Itching may be from irritation of fecal soiling, so clean yourself well with moistened tissues, *not dry toilet paper*, as it can injure sensitive skin. Do not wear clothes that are too tight or that itch, such as jeans, panty hose, and panties without cotton crotches. Itching can be caused from dry skin, so put baby lotion or vitamin A or E cream on and around the area to moisten the skin.

If there is a problem with the kidneys, the skin may react with minor irritations. Your whole body could feel like you were just attacked by a swarm of mosquitoes, or it could be irritated just in the rectal area. Nevertheless, work the reflex area to the kidneys, bladder, and the liver to stimulate healing circulation and flush out excess toxins. Also, drink additional water and fluids. When our family has any trouble with their kidneys, we take a K-B supplement and soon feel better.

Check for pinworms: If you notice these small thread-like parasites in your feces, you will need to get rid of them! In addition, they spread to others, so check your children and animals.

Several years ago when living in Hawaii, I noticed our outdoor cat, "Aloha," was getting very thin, later I noticed he had pinworms. We decided to give him some garlic, but he just spit it out. Then we opened a garlic oil capsule and mixed it with his food. The next day we did the same. The following day I took Aloha to the vet. All signs of pinworms had disappeared.

So I would suggest to anyone who suspects pinworms to eat some fresh garlic or take garlic oil capsules for a few days. Give garlic to everyone else in the family, too, including your dogs and cats. Pinworms hate garlic.

FOOT REFLEXOLOGY STOPPED HEMORRHOID PAIN IN MINUTES

I can tell you of many cases in which the pain of hemorrhoids was stopped in minutes. Moreover, the amazing fact is that all indications of the offending irritation vanished completely, never to return, even in some of the most severe cases.

Many patients have been relieved from the pain of hemorrhoids simply by pressing the reflex buttons around the heels of their feet. And others have used reflexology in their hands. Pressure to the corresponding reflex area will activate nature's healing life force into the congested veins in the rectum.

Although men do suffer with hemorrhoids, there are far more women afflicted with this painful and embarrassing complaint. The method that has given the quickest and most successful results in treating hemorrhoids is through the reflexes on the feet.

I am writing this chapter on hemorrhoids for all who have suffered in silence for many years. You will learn the best method for your particular case, and then be able to use it immediately if pain strikes.

REFLEXOLOGY HELPS PROLAPSED RECTUM

A prolapsed rectum is another condition that can cause untold agony. As a person gets older, this condition can get worse. The rectum is often badly swollen and very much inflamed and protrudes more and more. The benefit of reflexology is almost unbelievable for this serious condition. You will use the same method that you used for the hemorrhoid disorder, since this involves the same area.

When you use the techniques of reflexology, you are sending a healing power of nature to revive activity into the whole lower lumbar area.

I suffered from hemorrhoids for years and at times there was such excessive bleeding, I thought I would bleed to death. Many times, I would get up and work all night because the pain was so severe I couldn't lie down or sit still. I used every kind of ointment there was. The doctor didn't see anything seriously wrong. Since I wouldn't take drugs, I suffered in silence; piles are something you don't talk about.

How Reflexology Helped the Author

I was introduced to reflexology by a friend of my cousin who was visiting at her home. She was kind enough to give me a treatment. When she touched the reflexes to the hemorrhoids on my heels, I nearly went through the ceiling from the pain. She showed me how to find these buttons so I could work them myself. "You will never be bothered with hemorrhoids again if you work all of the tenderness out of the reflexes in this area," she promised. I thanked her, but can truthfully say that I doubted her word, even though I was amazed at the great feeling of stimulation I felt after the treatment. I did work the soreness out as she had instructed, "in just two or three days," and I have never had a recurrence of the disorder in these many years since. I also have never stopped using reflexology.

This encounter with reflexology led to my study of the amazing methods of this natural art of healing, and my study and research continue to this day.

CHAPTER 26

How Reflexology Can Help Your Heart

Heart disease, including certain circulatory disorders, is on the increase and results in more than one million deaths every year. Not only does it strike those who are in an advanced age, it is also a threat to many in the prime of life. But no matter what your health is today, you can improve it with nutritious meals, exercise, a positive attitude, and reflexology.

THE HEART AND HOW IT WORKS

The heart is a muscular organ with walls ranging from one-quarter to three-quarters of an inch in thickness. It is actually a pump that circulates the blood throughout the body. In the blood itself are the red corpuscles that take up and discharge oxygen during circulation. The whole process is continuous and takes about a minute for the blood to make a complete double circle through the body. Do you know that the heart muscle actually takes a rest after each beat, longer than the beat itself?

When you take your blood pressure, there is a high number (systolic pressure) which is when the heart is contracted, and a low number (diastolic pressure) which is slower because the heart is at ease, resting a moment before its next beat.

Tension, chest pain, perspiring, shortness of breath, and irregular heartbeat are a few symptoms of heart trouble. Studies show that women get nausea, jaw pain, and fatigue symptoms as well, while most men do not. The American Heart Association tells us that 24% of men and 42% of women will die within one year after having a heart attack. So you can see how significant using reflexology is to decrease anxiety in the body and release tension from the muscles. When the body relaxes, tautness decreases, and blood flow is enhanced to and from the heart.

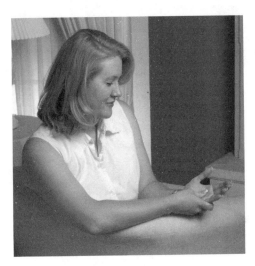

Photo 29: Position for working reflexes across the left hand which correspond to the heart, arteries, and veins. Stimulation to these reflexes helps boost nature's energy, giving the cardiovascular system a better chance to fight off heart disorders.

KEY REFLEXES FOR A HEALTHIER HEART

Notice in Photo 29 how the thumb of the right hand is pressed into the upper pad on the left palm. Remember that since the heart and its circulatory system extend over into the center of the body, you will press and work this whole area. Work the thumb clear across the palm, searching for tender spots as you go. When the sore spots are found, work them out, as they are telling you of congestion in the corresponding zone.

By looking at the Zone Chart, page 14, and Chart A, page 10, we see how the meridian zone lines one through five run throughout the areas of the heart and blood vessels. The circulation system carries oxygen-rich blood from the left side of the heart, around the body to all tissues, then returns oxygen-poor blood to the right side of the heart.

You can see, by *holding pressure* against the first through fifth fingers on the left hand, you will be calming the heart. When you use *stimulating movements* on reflexes to the heart, you are activating a vital life force into the left side of the body, thus sending oxygen-rich blood into the canals to help nature relieve congestion and revive glandular activity.

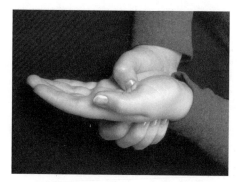

Photo 30: Position for placing fingers on back of hand, and thumb on palm side. Working the reflexes with this double-pressure encourages renewed circulation.

With your fingers on back of the hand and your thumb on the palm side, work the reflex areas simultaneously. (See Photo 30.) This double stimulation will improve circulation through' the heart and coronary arteries, as well as send vital energy to the lungs to help oxygenate your blood. Remember, some heart attacks are caused when a sticky blood clot, or blood with very little oxygen, totally closes the artery. So, do all you can to keep your circulation moving.

You have many internal systems that work together to protect your heart. Take your liver, for instance; it makes hundreds of compounds, including good cholesterol, that break down toxins in its chemical warehouse. You have just used the double stimulation on the heart reflex in your left hand. Now repeat this double-action on the liver reflex in your right hand. The liver and heart must safeguard each other to prevent heart disease.

Now let's highlight the other reflex areas you should concentrate on when using reflexology to help your heart. With your thumb, use a walking-technique and work across the chest, lung, and diaphragm reflexes, continuing to the outside of each hand, to the shoulder and arm reflex areas. This will send renewed circulation flowing through all five zones on both sides of your body.

You will want to work the kidney and bladder reflex areas on both hands to help filter waste from the blood system, and flush it out of the body. In addition, working up and down the spinal reflex area in zone one, from thumb to wrist, on each hand will stimulate renewed energy to the brain and spine. The brain stem controls body functions that occur naturally, such as your breathing and heartbeat. This reflex stimulation will help clear pathways so the functional nerve energies through the spinal cord have the power needed to reach all the organs that they serve, including your heart.

How Heart Pain Can Be Relieved with Reflexology

The heart can be aided with the reflex push buttons, no matter what the nature of the trouble is. I have treated heart complaints many times while we waited for a doctor to arrive, or until I was sure the afflicted person was out of danger and free from pain.

If there is pain in the chest or heart region, then the reflexes to the whole area should be massaged. If there are pains going along the arm and shoulder, which is characteristic of angina pectoris, then you will work the whole region, even up onto the little finger and around the outside of the left hand. Here we are trying to relieve tension. You may also use reflex clamps on all fingers of the left hand.

Many cases of death have been disclosed as heart failure, when the underlying causes are actually the poor condition of other glands that puts so much strain on the heart that it finally gives up.

People put an extra load on the heart by filling the lungs with nicotine and polluted air. They fail to eat the proper foods, yet wonder why they are stricken with a heart attack just when they were getting ready to enjoy life, not realizing that congestion has been accumulating for years in the veins around the heart and other organs.

How a Signal Forewarns of Heart Attack

While visiting my parents, I talked with their neighbor, Martin, a middle-aged man who had a history of heart attacks and was semi-invalid. I said to him one day, "If I tell you where to rub your feet for your heart, will you do it?" He looked at me rather oddly and said, "Oh, I suppose I would do anything if I thought it would help." I knew how doubtful he felt. "Can you reach your feet with your hands?" I asked. "Yes, I can still do that," he replied. So I told him, "You rub all around your little toe on the left foot, massaging especially on the upper pad just below the toe. Also do the same thing on your hands, working across the upper part of your left hand and around the little finger, and you may not have any more heart attacks."

Suddenly, his head came up and he really looked interested. "Why," he said in a surprised voice, "you know every time before I have an attack I noticed my little toe turns blue. I wondered about this, even mentioned it to my doctor, but no one knew the answer."

He said it started to turn blue several days before the attack. I told him, "If you had massaged it, maybe you would have prevented the attack." "I bet you are right," Martin said. "I will sure work on my little toe and fingers from now on."

Nature's barometer may warn of heart weakness: Could the blue color of this man's little toe be nature's warning signal, telling him that the heart was in need of help? I suggest watching this little barometer carefully if you are troubled with a heart condition. Work all the reflexes to the heart as directed in the preceding pages. The Magic Reflexer would also be useful here since it stimulates most of the glands in the whole body. As you squeeze and roll it in your hands, press its little fingers into all of the reflex buttons. Be sure to work the reflexes in both hands. The whole body may be out of harmony, and you are merely helping nature put it back in tune by working all the reflexes, giving her a chance to bring new life to the congested glands and dying cells in your body. Yes, health can be quickly and simply restored through reflexology.

How a Businessman Prevents Heart Attack

Mr. Scott told me about an experience he had not long ago in his office. "While I was working at my desk," he said, "I suddenly began to feel funny. My chest began to tighten up, I became nauseated, and pain started to travel up my left arm. I knew the signs of a heart attack, as I had one several years ago. As you know, I am an old reflexology enthusiast so I knew what to do.

"I just relaxed back in my chair without anyone noticing and started to massage the pad under my little finger on my left hand with the thumb of my right hand. I massaged clear across the hand to the reflexes near the web. I found the tender spot close to the stomach reflex and massaged it until it was no longer sore. I kept working on all of the heart reflexes for about a half hour, even though the pain had begun to subside as soon as I started to massage the reflexes in my hand.

"No one in the office was aware that anything was wrong and I was able to resume work in a normal manner, which I am

sure would not have been possible had I not known the value
of reflex massage. I have never had any trouble since, and I
know I never will so long as I use the magic of reflexology."

Let me give you a word of warning while we are on the subject of the heart. *Don't overdo!* Never overdo! Remember that your
heart is a muscle and when your outer muscles become flabby, so
do your inner muscles, like your heart. If your legs and arms are
very soft from lying around idle for a long time, you wouldn't try
to go out and run a foot race or play a game of tennis or ball just
because you felt good one day, would you? If you did, you would
probably have muscle spasms in your arms and legs.

The heart is a muscle, too, a big muscle in proportion to the
size of our body. In the average adult, the heart weighs from 9 to
11 ounces. If you overtax it with unusual exercise before giving it
a chance to build up strength after a long rest, it could very easily
have a muscle spasm, too—a heart attack!

This is what often happens when office workers who spend
most of their time sitting decide to go on a big adventuresome hike
up in the mountains, or suddenly dive into a strenuous exercise or
weight-lifting program. For instance, let me give you the experience Carl had.

Man Recovers Too Quickly

Carl came to me after suffering for months from a heart
condition. He took about three treatments from me in a period of seven days and felt so well he decided to go back to
work. He was sure he was well. I tried to tell him his heart was
still soft from his months of inactivity. I told him, "Give your
heart a chance to build up its strength. Wait awhile, give your
heart a chance." He felt so good he wouldn't listen and drove
over one hundred miles to ask for his old job back. He felt like
a new man. He walked all over the factory and up and down
many flights of stairs. He then walked up a long hill to his
parked car. This is when his heart began to protest. After that,
he went back into semi-invalidism.

He never came back to me. He had lost faith in this great
work that might have made him a healthy man for the rest of
his life if he had only listened, or used common sense.

So remember what happened to Carl. No matter how well you feel after working your reflexes, give your body time to renew its cells, and rebuild its muscles and strength.

Work Your Reflexes while in a Prone Position

Start out exercising slowly in a horizontal position while you are in bed or lie down on the floor. When you are lying down, all organs are on the same level with your heart, which helps it function with less exertion. This way blood is flowing along with gravity, not against it.

Wheel your Deluxe Hand & Foot Roller between your hands, lift it above your head, pump it up and down, and rotate it from side to side. Pass it from one hand to the other, and work the "massaging fingers" into reflexes on your palms and fingers (see Photo 12, page 48). Doing reflexology this way helps improves circulation quickly, without straining the heart to pump blood uphill. Some doctors do not recommend using reflexology for heart troubles. Always check with your doctors and follow their advice.

Exercising is very beneficial for your total well-being, but just take it easy at first. Take short walks, and maybe do a few knee bends each day to rebuild your strength. This way you will regain your energy gradually, and soon have the capacity, power, and good health to enjoy life at its best.

CHAPTER 27

How to Regulate Blood Pressure and Lower Cholesterol

Two problems for the cardiovascular system, which is comprised of the heart and blood vessels, are high blood pressure and bad cholesterol. If you eat animal fats, junk foods, or foods fried in grease, your cholesterol reading may become higher than it should be. If there is an obstruction of cholesterol plaque in your blood, your heart will have to work harder, and circulation through the vessels becomes strenuous. Thus, the blood pressure goes up, which can be very dangerous, as high blood pressure is a forerunner to heart problems and strokes.

HOW TO BRING DOWN HIGH BLOOD PRESSURE

High blood pressure is also referred to as *hypertension,* and when untreated can result in various health problems. Ringing in the ears, frequent nosebleeds, headache, fatigue, and dizziness are all symptoms of a blood pressure/hypertension imbalance.

Stress and tension affect blood pressure: When you are under stress, do you think your blood pressure's mounting? It probably is because stress can cause the artery walls to constrict, which makes your blood pressure rise. Anger, frustration, and negative thoughts also produce tensions. So if you start feeling uptight, try concentrating on positive thoughts and use reflexology pressure in the center of your left palm, while taking in a few slow, deep breaths. These simple precautions may help reduce anxiety and possibly save you from some serious health dilemmas.

There are hidden dangers when blood pressure is high: It can cause dangerous conditions that are debilitating, such as strokes, heart attacks, and kidney failure, even problems that can eventually lead to blindness. Therefore, you can see how important it is to return the blood vessels back to a normal state. Children should master reflexology at an early age, this way they can learn how to calm their nerves and hopefully avoid future health troubles.

HOW TO MANAGE LOW BLOOD PRESSURE

When an individual stands up too quickly and feels dizzy, it may be due to a reduced flow of blood going to the brain. The blood may not flow to the brain fast enough after you have been standing, sitting, or lying in one position for a long time. So, remember not to jump up or start walking away to quickly. Give your blood flow a chance to get to the brain before you move fast, and you may avoid the light-headed feeling.

If you feel dizzy, rub one hand over the other (like you're rubbing invisible lotion into dry skin) to wake up circulation. Do not forget the pituitary is your blood improvement center, so work this reflex in the pad of each thumb to strengthen brain energy. Give each thumb a deep workout.

Also, bend your ankles, knees, arms, and wrists before rising from your chair or bed. This will help rouse blood movement and give vessels time to contract, so that blood can be pumped to the brain, and then you can get up without dizziness. Using the Deluxe Hand & Foot Roller before getting up is a great way to stimulate circulation and help your body facilitate its own healing power.

How to Normalize Blood Pressure with Reflexology

Whether pressure is high or low, work the reflex areas that correspond to:

• The entire endocrine gland system, to balance and boost life force energies.
• The heart and arteries, to activate circulation.
• The digestive system, to help assimilate nutrients.

- The liver, kidney, and bladder, to manage fat and flush out toxins.
- The outside of each hand, if you suffer with shoulder or leg pain.
- The lungs and bronchial reflex area across both palms (take a few deep breaths for renewed oxygen flow), especially if you have trouble in breathing.

Reflexology helps flush out toxic fluids and promotes elimination of water from the body to help equalize blood pressure. Give yourself an *energizing* reflex workout to increase your stamina level, if you feel weak and tired. Alternatively, give yourself a *relaxing* reflex workout if you are uptight and need to reduce harmful stress and high blood pressure.

HOW TO MEASURE YOUR OWN BLOOD PRESSURE

You can test your own pulse-rate at home. The best time of day is in the morning. There are several places on the body that you can press to feel your pulse. However, the most convenient is on the thumb side of your left wrist. (See Photo 31.)

Place two or three fingertips in line with your thumb, and count the number of circulatory beats you feel within one minute. When you count your pulse, you are actually feeling a wave of blood as it is pumped from the heart and is now traveling along the arteries.

If you count between 60 to 70, it means that your heart is functioning well. However, if you count 80 beats or above in one minute, your heartbeat is very rapid and your heart is working too hard. This means it's time you make some serious changes in your diet, get more exercise (slowly at first), and use reflexology to improve your circula-

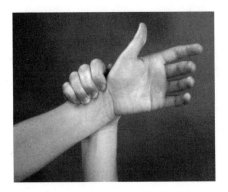

Photo 31: Position for conveniently taking your own pulse. Place fingertips in line with your thumb, and count the number of circulatory beats per minute, to determine the rate of your heartbeat.

tion. If your pulse rate remains high, consult your doctor to avoid any future illness.

Buddha Physician Could Feel Despair by Touching Pulse

I remember reading a true article written by the Dalai Lama, regarding one of Tibet's physicians, who would examine his patients by first reading their pulse. Although many doctors start their examinations by first taking the pulse, this physician could *feel* the health of the whole person—mentally, physically, and emotionally. He could perceive their emotions by just touching their pulse. Isn't this spectacular?

Yet, one sad story was about a young nun who had been tortured. When the Buddhist physician reached out with his hand and took her pulse, he became shocked. He could "feel despair from her pulse" and knew the depth and details of her terrible ordeals. He was sensitive to her needs; as tears ran down his cheeks, he made her some natural herbal healing formulas to help assist in her recuperation, and hopefully put an end to her suffering. By this story, we can see how powerful the pulse is to each person's well-being.

HOW TO REGULATE CHOLESTEROL

Keep a check on your cholesterol level. Do not let it go over 160, or you may be in danger of heart disease or possibly a stroke. Use reflexology and exercise to keep circulation moving. Lack of proper circulation and eating too much fat can cause high cholesterol in your blood.

There are two kinds of cholesterol. One is good; it is called *HDL* (high-density lipoprotein). This good component moves the cholesterol away from arteries and places it in the liver. Most of it rebuilds cell walls, and the rest is eliminated from the body.

The other is *LDL* (low-density lipoprotein), the bad cholesterol. The bad component forms a substance called *plaque* that clogs the coronary arteries. It resembles dried toothpaste. It is actually a white, waxy fat that gets thick and deposits in the main corridor of the arteries. It blocks off, and sometimes stops, the supply of blood traveling to the heart.

Helpful Tips to Lower Cholesterol Level

Make sure you are not overweight, as this can put you at risk. Exercise or walk every day to lower blood pressure and control weight.

• Learn the difference between saturated fat and unsaturated fats, then reduce saturated fats from your diet. They cause LDL, the "bad cholesterol," in your blood. Oils such as hydrogenated and partially hydrogenated are harmful fats that block circulation and can cause damage to the action of your heart. A few bad saturated fats are: palm, coconut, hydrogenated soybean, and cottonseed oils.

• Eat less fat and fewer cholesterol-rich foods and decrease your intake of sodium and carbohydrates.

• If you smoke, stop. It slows circulation and shuts off blood flow within the arteries.

• Sauerkraut (low-fat, low-salt in glass jars) and cultured yogurt are two good foods that lower cholesterol, boost immunity, and give your body the "friendly" bacteria it needs to stay healthy.

• Cook with the golden oils that cause HDL, the "good cholesterol," to form in your blood. These oils work with your body to lower bad cholesterol. A few golden oils are olive oil, flaxseed oil, and omega 3 fish oil. Those sold in dark glass are usually the best.

Udo Erasmus tells us in his book *Fats That Heal—Fats That Kill* of Dr. Johanna Budwig's discovery of the healing powers of combining protein-rich cottage cheese (or quark) with raw flaxseed oil. The doctor has researched and found that together these two foods replenish electrical energy to the entire physiological condition of the body. Only when combined with each other, the essential fatty acids and rich proteins work to assist the body's microorganisms to take up oxygen. The blending of these two foods help rebuild new brain, nerve, and tissue cells, as well as heal worn-out muscles.

Dr. Budwig's research shows flaxseed oil combined with certain proteins can help the body reduce cholesterol levels, normalize blood pressure levels, and build up the immune system. Studies also show increased metabolism and anti-tumor activity, even repression of cancer cell growth.

Give yourself a little test if you think you may be consuming too much fat. After your next bowel movement, check the toilet paper to see if waste matter is smeared with grease. Dr. Marsh Morrison tells us if you have eaten a lot of fatty foods, the stool will smear on the tissue, and you will have a harder time cleaning yourself. Once you improve your diet and stop eating fatty or oily meals, you will notice a cleaner bowel movement and less toilet tissue will be needed.

HOW TO CORRECT CIRCULATORY PROBLEMS

Arteriosclerosis and atherosclerosis occur when blood flow from the arteries to the heart is blocked, causing the circulatory system to slow down. You can help free up these blockages by improving your circulation with reflexology and exercising as able. You can also cut down on your fat intake and lower your cholesterol level to correct slow-flowing circulation.

Poor circulation can leave you with cold hands and feet, muscle cramps, and respiratory troubles. Slow circulation can also cause blurred vision, lung, heart, or artery degeneration, and mental problems.

You must keep your circulation moving. Do not allow yourself to become sluggish. Good circulation will help the body detoxify itself, and getting rid of old toxins is very important to your health.

Reflexology encourages healthy circulation. It is easy to use and will help invigorate your body's lymphatic and circulatory systems, as well as help oxygenate the blood.

KEY REFLEX POINTS TO HELP IMPROVE CIRCULATION

Work the heart reflex area on your left hand, and all the lymph gland reflex points to help regulate your blood pressure. (See Charts B and C.) Work the pituitary gland reflex in both thumbs. This gland is the leader of the endocrine glands, which secretes chemical hormones into the bloodstream helping to regulate all the other systems. Check all endocrine gland reflexes for tenderness.

Work across the upper part of the palm of each hand to send energy to your lungs. While working on the lung reflex, take a few deep breaths. Now with your thumb and index finger, work the Magical V on each hand. (See Photos 7 and 58.)

Work across the entire digestive system, giving extra attention to the large and small intestine reflexes on each hand. Keep your colon clean by eating vegetables and fiber cereals. Constipation and colon toxicity will make your metabolism sluggish and cause poor circulation.

Work the large reflex area to your liver, on the right hand. The liver works so hard it produces heat that warms the blood. As the heated blood circulates, it keeps the whole body warm.

Rotate the Deluxe Hand & Foot Roller between your hands quickly to renew circulation movement (see Photo 32). Use the same roller under your feet. Place your left foot on top of the roller and *briskly* move it back-and-forth over the roller, so that all the little roller fingers press into the reflex points on the bottom of your foot. Repeat with your right foot. This will promote circulation throughout the whole body and encourage warmer blood flow.

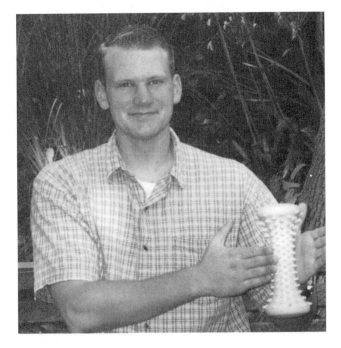

Photo 32:
Place the Deluxe Hand & Foot Roller between hands and *quickly* roll it back and forth. This encourages renewed circulation throughout all energy zones and promotes the body's self-healing powers.

How Dr. Shute cures heart patients: You may know the wonderful results Dr. Wilfrid E. Shute of the Shute Foundation, London, Canada has obtained with heart patients by using Vitamin E in his hospital. Vitamin E improves oxygen supply and circulation. The doctor tells us that this vitamin helps reduce cholesterol, saturated fats, and even helps in reducing scar tissue after a heart attack. Vitamins combined with exercise, a nutritious diet, and reflexology should put the rate of death from heart disease down at the bottom of the "dangerous health problems" list.

Reflexology Helps Friends in the Caribbean Islands

Dear Mrs. Carter:

Just a few lines to let you know that receiving your book on "reflexology" was the answer to my prayers.

I am a man 65 years old and I was suffering with pains and aches all over. Ever since I applied reflexology, I feel like a new man: Thanks to you. I have been treating friends of mine and I have recommended your book, if they want to follow their own treatments.

During my vacation, I went to the Caribbean Islands. In Puerto Rico, I met a man who told me that two of the fingers on his left hand had no circulation and were numb. He was afraid to wear his expensive rings for fear that they might drop off and he would not know about it. I gave him a reflex treatment and to his surprise and mine, his fingers were okay.

In the Dominican Republic, we visited a family of friends and met a lady who was suffering from pains all over the right side of her head, neck, and shoulder. She said, "Sometimes the pain goes down to the leg." I offered to give her right side a treatment which she accepted. We went away and when we returned three hours later we stopped to inquire if the treatment had done anything for her. And the answer I got was that she grabbed me, hugged, and kissed me.

To tell you the truth, Mrs. Carter, they made me feel like a big shot. One drawback is the senoritas thought that I was the man they had been waiting for and proposed marriage to me.

Well, Mrs. Carter, may the Good Lord bless you and I beg to remain your healthful friend.

C.G.

CHAPTER 28

How to Use Reflexology for a Stroke

If you have had a stroke, or are in danger of having one, reflexology can be your salvation. Many strokes are caused by diminished circulation to the brain, thus the brain suffers from a lack of oxygen. Since the reflexes to the head are located mainly in the area of the thumbs, this is where you will concentrate your work. Use the press-and-rotate method on the pads, all around the sides, and on top of both thumbs.

Then work the same portion of all fingers, as they also contain reflexes that correspond to the brain. If you've had a stroke, you are searching for a tender spot, and when you find it, you will focus on working this reflex point, very gently at first. When you find an extremely tender spot in the thumb, it is indicative of a reflex to brain trouble. This could be a sign of brain damage caused by the stroke. You should also work the reflexes in your second and third fingers. Working the reflexes to the brain helps control the central nervous system.

Work the pituitary reflex in the end of each thumb and all the other endocrine system reflexes (see Chapter 6) along with the reflexes to the spinal area, which extend down the thumb to the wrist on each hand. Many nerves emerge from the brain and spinal cord that control motor function. The spinal cord, which is an extension of the brain, transports information to and from your organs, glands, muscles, and nerves.

Work the webbing of the Magical V, as explained on page 34, and the solar plexus and diaphragm in the center of each hand, as shown in Photo 45 on page 261. This is an energy network that will be helpful in balancing the nervous system functions.

If damage affects one side of the head, then go to the fourth and fifth fingers, working all around them, until you find a sore spot, then apply reflex pressure to it. Working reflex areas in fingers on both hands is important to balance and correct stroke damage. (Work feet also for best results.)

The Magic Reflexer works deeply into the reflex areas at the end of the thumb and fingers. (See Photo 22, page 132.) You can exert pressure on the reflexes with good advantage, holding the pressure from five to twenty minutes.

Work each thumb, finger, and along the spinal reflex area to stimulate vital energy, to promote blood flow to the brain. Alternatively, you can also stimulate blood flow by using the Deluxe Hand & Foot Roller, as explained in Chapter 5.

How to Prevent a Stroke

The biggest causes of a stroke are stress, insufficient circulation from lack of exercise, and eating fatty foods that plug the arteries. You can reduce the risk of a stroke by using reflexology to reduce tension, exercising your body, and eating many fresh fruits, vegetables, and grains for fiber. Also, remember to avoid salty and fatty foods.

An unhealthy heart and overexertion are two other causes of stroke. So when starting an exercise regimen, go slowly at first and gradually add to your routine as you become physically stronger.

Since high blood pressure increases the risk of strokes, you will want to concentrate on the reflexes to the liver on the right hand. (See Photo 35, page 213.) Also, work the reflex to the heart on the left hand. (See Photo 29, page 184.) Also, the reflexes to the pituitary gland that are located in the pad of each thumb, as shown on Chart B (page 11) and in Photo 4 (page 30).

Follow the health rules of bringing down blood pressure, and work the reflex areas described within Chapter 27 for lowering cholesterol and correcting circulation.

How to Use Reflexology After a Stroke

After a stroke, there may be several lost capabilities; however, in many cases skill and aptitude can be reacquired over a period of time. A stroke affects the central nervous system in the brain, so you will work the reflexes in the thumbs and fingers that correspond to the brain. (Each hemisphere of the brain controls the *opposite* side of the body. If a stroke were in the right side of the brain, the left side of the body would suffer the trauma.) In this situation, give extra attention to the thumb and fingers on the *opposite* side of the body that suffers paralysis.

Keep in mind that working reflexes in the left hand will send energy to the corresponding left side of the brain, and those in the right hand correspond to the right side of the brain. Recovery will depend on the reflex receiver's attitude and the extent of brain damage from the stroke.

Eating well helps speed recovery, so eat nutritious meals such as those that include fish and beans, and check with the doctor regarding some helpful supplements while you recuperate, such as Vitamins E and C, as they help speed the healing process.

We can see that since a stroke is caused by some malfunction of the body, it is so important to treat all reflexes to help stimulate the flow of life force energy to every gland and organ. This helps nature restore the whole body back to its natural balance and harmony with the universe.

Remember, when one instrument is out of tunes it causes the whole orchestra to be out of harmony, and, like a great orchestra, when one of your glands is malfunctioning, your health goes into a rasping discord.

So, never neglect working all of the reflexes at least two times a week when you are treating a certain illness or just for general health reasons.

Although I helped many people recover from strokes, I would like to include here reports from others who have had success with this method of treatment after using the directions as given in my book on foot reflexology. The treatment is as effective with hand reflex therapy, in most cases.

Stroke Victim Helped by Reflexology

My wife had a stroke several years ago but her progress was very slow and doctors didn't seem to do anything about it. About six weeks ago I purchased your book on Foot Reflexology, and started to give my wife treatments. To our surprise, it worked miracles, and in this short time she is almost back to normal and still improving. The doctors are dumbfounded and can't figure it out. I haven't told them, as they would only ridicule it.

Mr. A.

How a Brain-Damaged Victim Recovers

I am more convinced than ever that reflexology really works. I just finished a case where I had an occasion to use this type of therapy.

My patient was a cardiac arrest and was comatose for three days. She also had brain damage which affected her equilibrium. The doctors said she would not walk for at least six months, if ever. She had uremic poisoning and other complications. The doctor told me I could give her reflexology. The first week I gave her two treatments, and the very second day I observed an almost immediate response. Within three weeks, she was walking with help, and in one month she was walking alone and was discharged from the hospital. I continued treating her at home for a few weeks, twice a week. She is now as good as ever, and is out working in her garden every day.

Mrs. H.

A Miracle Happened Before My Very Eyes

Dear Mrs. Carter,

Something happened at the Penang Medical Center that I would like to share with you. The doctors and specialist almost gave up hope on Mr. Loo Leong Kee (77 years old then). He was suffering from a very severe stroke. His arteries were narrowing and the doctors sounded an alarm. "He can die any moment." Mr. Loo was in a coma. His niece rang me up and asked me whether reflexology could help. She said that all the medications applied didn't seem to bring down his blood pressure. So I told her, though I have done more than 15 cases of stroke, not one of them measures up to this kind. Anyway, I told her that I would give it a try. Deep in my heart, I thought it was a "mission impossible." But my policy is, "never give up the ship."

So the following day, I went to the Medical Center. Mr. Loo was on oxygen. I shifted his blanket aside and I chose the right foot first, because the liver is on the right foot. I gave him a very thorough treatment, then punctuated it with a bit of rejuvenation, by circling the feet around, from the left to right, and then right to left in order to release tension. Then, I concentrated on the magic button . . . the liver. This is the magic of Mildred Carter.

That was perhaps the turning point. The liver is the one that brings down the cholesterol level. I firmly believe that the liver is the real culprit of high blood pressure. I then applied the same procedure to the left foot, and after tuning the endocrine glands, I spent some time on the heart reflexes and the urinary tract. After finishing both feet, I went to the hand reflexes. Worked each hand for seven minutes, concentrating on the urinary tract, but stimulating all reflex areas.

On the second visit, I asked his brother how was the blood pressure. He said, "It has gone done from 220/120 to 170/100, a great improvement." That gave me an added inspiration. And on the third day after my reflex work, Mr. Loo began to open his eyes, looking as if he had returned from outer space. A miracle happened before my very eyes. His blood pressure returned to normal 150/90 and it remained stable for the rest of the week. Within a month, he could walk with the aid of a walking frame. Mr. Loo is doing fine now, and is 81 years old today. Wishing you and Tammy great happiness and the best of health.

Yours sincerely,

Mr. B.C., Penang

CHAPTER 29

Helping the Kidneys and Bladder with Reflexology

Your kidneys are certainly a great example of ingenuity. They are two little filtering systems, located behind the abdomen, one on each side of the spine. Millions of very small blood vessels make up the kidneys. All blood goes through the kidneys, which clean out impurities and then return it to the heart. The kidneys flush out old toxins and waste materials mixed with water through hollow tubes called *ureters*. The liquid waste travels into the bladder, and then is eliminated as urine.

Sometimes people donate one of their kidneys to another person whose own kidneys have stopped functioning. No one can live without at least one kidney to filter poison out of the body. I wonder how many such operations might be avoided if reflexology was used to help nature reactivate circulation of the vital life force back into these malfunctioning organs. It would do no harm to give reflexology a chance before drastic measures are taken.

REVITALIZE YOUR KIDNEYS WITH REFLEXOLOGY

Looking at Chart A on page 10, you can see that the kidneys are located on each side of the spine. Notice in Chart B (page 11) there is a reflex for the left kidney in the palm of the left hand, and a reflex for the right kidney, in the right hand. In Photo 33, page 204, you can see how the right thumb is placed in the left hand over the left kidney reflex.

Work this area by using a press-and-rotate method on the reflex. If the kidneys are badly affected, work this reflex point for only a few seconds the first few times. You do not want to overwork the urinary tract at first, as too much toxic waste draining from the system all at once could make you feel ill.

If you look at Charts D and E (pages 13 and 14), you will see that the kidneys are located within zones two and three. You can help in their fight for life by working the reflexes along fingers two and three. Since we are going to need all the stimulation we can get to reactivate the healing forces back into these organs, you might also work on the kidney and urinary reflexes in the feet.

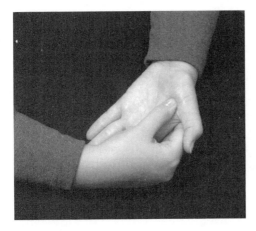

Photo 33: Position for working the left kidney and adrenal gland reflex on the left hand. Reverse hands and then work the right kidney and adrenal reflex on the right hand.

Nature's tendency is to restore all normal conditions in the body when we give her the necessary help by stimulating circulation of the vital life force with reflexology. When the Magic Reflexer is used in this area, the kidney reflexes will automatically get their share of stimulation. Remember, if you have a kidney problem, do not overwork its reflex area. You can work it more as the kidney is on its way to recovery.

To stimulate better kidney function, give a complete reflexology workout to renew circulation throughout the whole body. It is important to work the pituitary gland reflex in each thumb, as it secretes *vasopressin*, a hormone that regulates the water balance in the kidneys. You should work the reflexes to the adrenals and urinary system at least twice a week to help the body flush out accumulated impurities and prevent kidney troubles.

HOW TO TEST FOR KIDNEY WEAKNESS

Test the kidney reflex area in each hand. Press the kidney reflex in the left and then the right hand. If it is tender on either side, you will know there is not enough circulation getting to the kidney, corresponding to this tender reflex.

Test the kidney reflex on each foot. The kidney reflex in the foot is located on the sole, just above the waistline, and a little in from the instep, on each foot. Refer to my book *Healing Yourself with Foot Reflexology* for exact reflex location. If there is tenderness here, your kidneys may be in a weakened condition.

When the kidneys are in trouble, they send a dull ache into the lower lumbar. If your kidneys are ill, you may notice a faint discomfort in the lower back when you pick up a slightly heavy item. You may also feel a dull pain radiate through the kidneys when you jog, jump, or stomp your feet.

How to use your fists to test kidneys: Your kidneys lie directly behind the small of your back on either side of the spine. You can determine the health of each kidney by folding your fingers inward to make two fists and placing both hands behind your back, just above the waistline. Gently tap on the soft spots. If this area is tender when you tap it with your knuckles, your kidneys are most likely weak and need some serious reflexology attention.

How to help your kidneys with body reflexology: First rub your hands together energetically, as this will promote energy into the palms and fingers. Stand with your shoulders slightly bent forward. Place hands on your hips, with fingers toward naval, and thumbs pointing toward the spine. Move thumbs approximately two or three inches from the spine and two or three inches above the waistline. Search for the soft area in the small of your back. Using your thumbs or knuckles, work over the kidneys with a circular pressing motion. This will create a soothing heat from the friction and help reduce pain.

Gently tapping over the kidneys with your fists will stimulate healing circulation to strengthen and energize them, helping them to heal and function properly.

Temporarily ease pain by taking a nice warm bath to increase blood flow and loosen muscles around the kidney area. You can put a little Epsom salts in the water to enhance muscle relaxation.

For additional relief, apply Tea Tree Ointment or Kwan loong Oil over the lower back to reduce muscular tension and back pain.

FAULTY KIDNEYS CAN CAUSE VARIOUS HEALTH TROUBLES

Defective kidneys can cause a variety of health problems, such as chronic headaches, urinary infections, kidney stones, eye weakness, and impotent sex glands. In treating these conditions with reflexology, you will concentrate on the endocrine system (see Chapter 6) and the entire urinary tract.

Work back and forth between the bladder and adrenal gland reflex on each hand to relax tension, so nature can eliminate kidney troubles and other congestion through normal muscular contractions. Always be sure to work the reflexes in both hands; never unbalance nature by leaving one side untuned.

Work the reflex to and around the lower spine, to relax tense muscles and help release pressure from any pinched nerves that might be blocking circulation to these precious organs.

Kidney stones are caused when mineral deposits (mostly calcium) build up in the kidneys. These crystals need liquid to float. If there is not enough fluid, the sharp edges stick and build up, making it hard for them to dissolve and pass through the system. So you can see why it is so necessary to drink enough natural juices and quality water to dilute your urine and reduce the concentration of uric acid. Flush your kidneys every day to keep your urinary system clean.

If you are experiencing pain radiating from the upper part of your back to the lower stomach area, with chills, fever, and frequent urination containing pus and blood, there is most likely an infected stone in the urinary tract, and you will need medical attention.

Kidney failure is when the kidneys do not function normally. They cannot clean the blood properly and this causes a chemical imbalance and poisonous fluid back-up in the body. If you experience painful kidney reflexes and nausea, fever, severe pain, or vomiting, see your doctor.

Man Passes Stone in Ten Minutes

Dear Mrs. Carter,

I have to write and tell you what happened to me after I received your book. I started to use the directions about massaging the reflexes in my feet, and in about ten minutes I went to the bathroom and passed a stone. It was big enough to make a noise when it hit the water. I didn't even know I had any stones. I guess you know what I think of your wonderful book. I feel great thanks to you.

W.M., Kansas City, Mo.

Health tips: As we know, the urinary system cleans our blood, but we also need to remember that when blood is filled with toxic poison, it is really hard for the kidneys to clean it all. Some dirty blood may return into the circulation system, and when this happens, it is harmful to the body. So let us not forget, that what we eat is very valuable to our health.

Avoid eating salty, fatty, and sweet foods, as they offer your body no nutrition, but instead cause acid to form and create too much waste. Tomatoes also cause a lot of acid, so avoid them. Instead, eat plenty of onions, garlic, asparagus, parsley, and celery, with multi-grains, as these foods help the body heal.

Drink fresh juice, or eat fruit, such as watermelon, cantaloupe, apples, or peaches. Fruits have several ounces of extremely nutritious liquid in them, also helpful in flushing out and eliminating toxic waste. Good clean quality or distilled water is also going to help improve the health of your kidneys and urinary performance.

A well-known drink for kidney cleansing is two tablespoons raw apple cider vinegar and one tablespoon honey (or fresh lemon juice and honey) mixed into warm water. Drink this mixture for several days in the morning before your meal. Vinegar is a good "flush," and honey has healing properties that replenish energy.

During the day, drink lots of other high-quality or freshly squeezed juices, such as cranberry or apple. Drink warm soup broth without any salt as often as possible to help flush out built-up minerals. K-B is a wonderful urinary flush supplement made of juniper berries, parsley, and other herbs; it is a very good herbal diuretic.

Malfunctioning kidneys also affect eyes, bladder, and sex glands. So remember, when you are working the reflex to the kidneys, you are also strengthening the health of your eyesight and bladder, in addition to activating the sex glands.

REFLEXOLOGY FOR BLADDER TROUBLES

By relaxing tension and breaking up congestion with reflexology, I have had many wonderful results in helping cases of bladder troubles. Bladder infections often cause a frequent urge to urinate, along with a stinging, burning pain when you come to the end of emptying your bladder. There may be frequent, painful, or difficult urination, with cloudy urine that has a bad odor. The function of the urinary system is to cleanse the blood, but if you notice blood in your urine, you should consult your doctor.

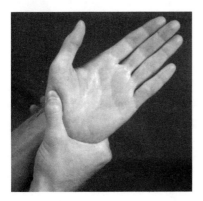

Photo 34: Position for working the reflex to the bladder and lower lumbar area, on the left hand. To reactivate and balance Nature's free flow of self-healing energy, work reflexes on both hands.

You have already located the bladder and its reflexes on the charts in the front of this book, but let us refer back to Chart B (page 11). Notice that the reflexes to the bladder are located in the lower part of each hand. Now look at Photo 34 and review the position of the thumb on this area. If the bladder is congested or affected in any way, you will find these reflexes quite tender. Work this with the press-and-rotate motion of your thumb. Continue to the wrist, on the lower lumbar reflexes. Stimulation on these reflexes allows normal circulation to flow through the cells as nature intended.

Reflex Help for the Urinary System

First give a complete reflex workout to tune up all systems, then double back and work from the bladder, along the urethra tube, to the kidney reflex. Turn your hands and follow this path back to the bladder reflex. (See Photo 59, page 284.)

Another technique is to place your thumb on the bladder reflex in your palm and fold the index finger and other fingers onto the backside of the hand, just opposite the thumb. Use a press-and-pull technique here. (See Illustration 4 on page 22.) Repeat on the other hand.

Work the reflex areas to the endocrine glands: It is imperative to keep these hormone glands functioning well, as they work in conjunction with the urinary system. If you are female, give the reflex to these glands special attention around your menstrual time. Also, women should remove tampons, diaphragms, or any other product that may be aggravating a bladder infection.

Reflex the lower abdominal area: Next, you will work up and down the spinal reflex area, concentrating on the lower spine reflex and the muscles that surround it. Work over the reflex area of the abdomen, intestines, and colon on both hands to encourage bowel movements. If constipated, you will feel additional pressure on the bladder, kidneys, and in your lower back.

Since the bladder is in the center of your body, Reflex Clamps on fingers one, two, and three can also be very beneficial in helping nature relax and heal congestion in the bladder area. In addition, the Magic Reflexer is safe and easy to use. As you turn it in your hand, it will activate the thymus, spleen, and lymph node reflexes to strengthen your immune system activities, which help fight off infections.

Avoid eating acid-forming foods like tomatoes, sodas, sweets, and junk foods. Do not neglect to see your naturopath or doctor if the infection continues, as it might be of a more serious nature, one that needs medical attention.

How Bedwetting Can Be Helped with Reflexology

When children, or seniors, wet the bed, it could be from weak organs, or it could be from a compressed nerve, or an allergic contraction within the bladder.

We must cope with this situation in a very patient manner, as bedwetting does not happen on purpose. Proper circulation is very important, so reflex over both hands and up forearms. Work reflexes to the pituitary gland to regulate water balance in the kidneys. Work up and down the spinal reflex area, and awaken all reflexes to the urinary system.

Drink no water or juices before going to bed. If thirsty, eat a small stalk of celery to curb the dry feeling, and satisfy the need for salt.

Look also to other glands that often are the real cause of bladder trouble. If you find tender reflexes in any area of the hands or feet, they are sending out a cry for help, so *if the reflex hurts, work the tenderness out.*

Reflexologist from India Gives History of Healings

Mr. Thj, a very successful reflexologist in Arizona, studied reflexology in India and has a unique and successful way of working the reflexes to help nature promote healing of malfunctioning parts of the body. He was aided back to walking after being told that he would never walk again. He was also helped to better vision by the use of reflexology.

I will let Mr. Thj tell you in his own words how he helped one lady.

"The other night I was treating a lady who has had several treatments, only on this particular night she had obtained a nasty cut from a rose thorn. I worked all around it on the right foot, then I went to the pituitary reflex on the left foot. After a second or two I asked her to wet her finger with saliva from her own mouth and put it on the cut on her right foot. Then I continued the treatment. After the treatment I asked her to look at the sore. To her amazement there was nothing there but a red mark, like those left when you peel a scab from an old cut."

Mrs. Thj adds—"Reflexology has helped me with a bladder problem (since childhood) which was very embarrassing, to say the least. Also reflexology has rid me of the pain in my bunion, which I thought would be with me to the grave. It hurt 24 hours a day."

CHAPTER 30

How to Use Reflexology to Help the Liver

The liver is your largest organ and is of vital importance to the well-being of your entire body. It is part of the digestive system, which receives food-rich blood from the small intestine, breaks it down, mixes it with oxygen-rich blood, and then sends the processed blood to the heart.

Resting behind the right lower ribs, it reaches across the chest to the stomach. It weighs from three to four pounds, is approximately the size of a football (smaller in small people), and has roughly five hundred jobs to perform. So you can see the importance of giving this busy organ all the help it needs.

Our liver works so hard digesting food and fats with the secretion of bile, assisting intestinal actions, regulating blood sugar levels and so on, that it produces heat, which warms the blood and helps keep our whole body warm.

THE LIVER IS YOUR BODY'S HIGH-TECH LABORATORY AND STOREHOUSE

It cleans the blood: When the liver receives the food-filled blood, it first cleans it of toxic substances and detoxifies poisons such as nicotine, alcohol, drugs, and chemical preservatives. Then it flushes them out through the kidneys.

Is a storage center: The liver takes in many vitamins from the foods we eat, and even stores a few for later, then releases them as needed by the body. It stores Vitamin A to help our vision, B vitamins and iron which make our red blood cells, and Vitamin D, needed for healthy bones and teeth.

Manufactures and secretes bile: Bile is a green liquid necessary for digestion. It helps absorb many vitamins and minerals from the food you eat and helps prevent constipation. The gall bladder stores bile until it's needed, then releases it into the duodenum to keep your body nourished and functioning well.

Breaks down fat: If you are overweight and do not understand why, it may be due to an overworked liver. What you eat is very important to the health of your liver. If you have a poor diet that includes junk foods, lots of fats, white flour, or sugar products, then your liver is overburdened. As it works hard, trying to remove poisons from the blood, you will start feeling tired. Moreover, it will not be long before you notice that you are gaining weight.

When you overeat, your liver has a surplus of food. It uses some, and the rest it converts to fatty tissues and stores them throughout the body. To get well, you must improve your diet. Once the liver is set free of its heavy work schedule (storing fat cells), it will return to its original job of purifying your blood, flushing out fats, improving your metabolism, and giving you renewed energy. One woman told me that by working the reflex to her liver everyday, she has noticed a decrease in cellulite and firmer thighs.

Fatty acids and sugar molecules are reorganized in the liver. Glycogen (sugar from converted nutrients) is taken out of the blood and held in storage for future use. When the body needs it, the liver returns it as glucose (blood sugar) to the bloodstream.

The liver is a blood purifier that removes such waste products as worn-out red blood cells, hormones, and toxic substances. It not only manufactures coagulants, which keep you from bleeding to death, but also anticoagulants that keep your blood from thickening dangerously in the arteries.

This interesting and indispensable organ has the power to rebuild itself if given a chance, even after a large part of it has been destroyed by disease. It is not possible to go into detail about the liver's numerous functions, but you can see that this important health-builder needs all the stimulation it can get in order to keep the body functioning in perfect order.

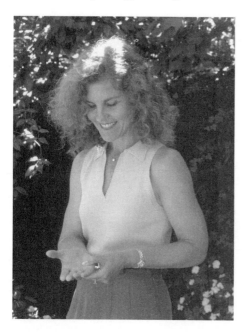

Photo 35: Position for working the reflex area to the incredible liver. The liver is responsible for over 500 functions, one of which helps prevent constipation; another helps break down fats.

WORKING REFLEXES TO HELP THE LIVER HEAL ITSELF

As we just mentioned, the liver has extraordinary healing qualities; when one part is damaged, it can grow new cells to rebuild itself. So, let us help with the healing power of reflexology. As you can see from Chart B on page 11, the reflexes to the liver are rather crowded within a comparatively small area of the hand. Study the chart for the exact location. Remember that the liver is located primarily on the right side of the body, so the reflex area is on the right hand.

Using the side or tip of your left thumb, press with a rolling motion across the right hand with a criss-cross technique. This means to work across the hand, turn, and work back. It is even more beneficial if you work up into the reflex of the lungs while working the liver. Also, work the reflex to the heart on the left hand. Make sure the energy extends through these divisions, as they are all interrelated.

Work this whole area *firmly* to restore natural circulation. Check for any tender spots that might give you a warning signal that the liver has become sluggish and needs your life-giving help. Work any sore reflexes and send renewed vitality and life force to this vital organ. Do not be afraid to work a large area here. Remember that the liver is the largest organ in the body, so its reflex area in the hand is also very large.

If you find soreness in the liver reflex, you can expect several different reactions from the treatment. Some people become temporarily lightheaded. Others feel tired and listless after the first workout session, so if your body needs to relax, take a rest. One of my patients had a dozen bowel movements in one day after his second reflex treatment. If this happens to you, do not worry; it is only nature doing her long-delayed house cleaning. You will feel much better when the cleaning job is completed.

Give a complete reflex workout to all zones in both hands to balance the body and help stimulate the flow of blood and lymph through the liver. Work up into the lungs and heart area to make sure the energy extends through all zones, as they are all interrelated. Do some deep breathing exercises to encourage oxygen-rich blood into your liver.

When the liver is sluggish, the body will feel very tired and congested. Then you know it's time to work the reflex area to all the endocrine glands for increased energy. Also, work the reflex area from the upper-mid part of both hands, down to the inside of the wrist. This will correspond to your urinary and digestive systems and help the body flush out toxins. Give extra attention to the kidney reflex on both hands; the kidneys must function correctly in order for the liver to perform accurately.

If you feel nauseous, it may be because the liver is malfunctioning. Look for tender spots in the Magical V reflex area, between the thumb and index finger of the right hand. (See Photo 7, page 33.) Also, search in the webbing between the other fingers, checking for sore spots in all zones. Now work the third and fourth zones on your right forearm, about two inches from the wrist, as the corresponding location involves the hepatic artery, which brings renewed oxygen-rich blood to the liver.

If your hands are yellow or flushed, it may indicate trouble with the liver. Follow directions for overcoming liver trouble and search out all sore spots in the liver reflex area.

How Finger Squeezing Benefits the Liver

Now we will learn how to squeeze certain fingers that will not only work as an anesthetic if there is pain, but will help in the healing process as well. Concentrating on the right hand, let us move up to the first joint of the four fingers, fingers 2, 3, 4, and 5. See the Zone Chart on page 14. Press these fingers thoroughly on the sides, and then press the front and back of each finger. (See Photos 5 and 6, page 32.)

If you need assistance, the reflex clamps may be applied for a few minutes to give a steady pressure on these reflexes. They will not only act to minimize pain, but also to stimulate the electric life forces of nature to heal the areas to which the reflexes are connected. If your hands feel sore or tired, the Hand Probe or Magic Reflexer are both very good self-help tools and work well to stimulate this large reflex area.

Use a reflex comb for extra stimulation to liver: You can use the comb technique in working reflexes to the liver, as well as many other glands, as explained in Chapter 5. Taking the sturdy comb in the right hand and pressing the ends of the four fingers on the teeth of the comb will help stimulate the liver into new life. (See Photo 61, page 285.) You may also press the comb into this reflex area on the palm, by turning the comb over with the teeth down and using fingers to apply pressure, for an extra stimulus.

Symptoms from a Neglected Liver

If you notice the whites of your eyes, tongue, and skin have a yellow color to them, it could be your liver calling out for help, warning you of an infection or blockage. If your urine or bile is dark in color, your gall bladder may also need help. These symptoms could mean jaundice, hepatitis, or a tumor. Dark bile is often caused when taking a supplement with high amounts of iron. In this case, cut back on your iron intake. Seek medical help if needed.

Tips for a Healthy Liver

Do not allow yourself to become overweight. Use reflexology and get lots of exercise. Walking is good for the health of your entire body and helps with circulation. Eat several small meals throughout the day for effective digestion, not large heavy meals at one time. Poor food choices and overeating will cause liver malfunction.

Foods that can help your liver and your body are fresh vegetables. Eat them raw, steamed, or make fresh juices. Most are high in Vitamin A and C, which helps the body rebuild new liver cells and tissues. Milk thistle tea is excellent help for rebuilding tissues, and garlic is very good for the liver, as it helps detoxify the bloodstream. Avoid a diet that causes constipation, such as sugar, grease, and animal fats. These products can cause poor digestion, a sluggish liver, and gallstones.

A two- or three-day internal body wash with little or no solid food will help rinse out your system. During this event, you will want to drink lots of fresh juice several times each day and extra water to help stimulate digestive enzymes and flush out built-up fats and cholesterol. Coenzyme Q-10 helps the liver receive more oxygen. Follow directions on the bottle. Fresh applesauce is good fiber and very beneficial for the liver.

KEY REFLEXES FOR GALL BLADDER TROUBLE

Preventing gallstones should be a priority in your life. Severe pain in the top right side of the abdomen—along with fever, vomiting, and nausea—can be the signal of an inflamed gall bladder. Cholesterol from too much fatty food can crystallize in bile fluid and form tiny sores that block the bile passageway.

Using reflexology can encourage circulation to the gall bladder and boost your immune system. With your thumb or a self-help tool, work back and forth across the liver and gall bladder reflex area on your right palm. Also concentrate on the reflexes to the urinary and digestive system. Work up and down the spinal reflex area, and give both hands a good reflex workout to help your body naturally regain a healthy liver and gall bladder.

Traveler Uses Steering Wheel to Relieve Liver Complaints

I woke up this morning with a dull ache in the region of my liver and gall bladder, accompanied by a headache, both of which I attributed to having overeaten a lot of rich foods at a late dinner party last night. I had an early appointment some ten miles from home, and I wondered if it was safe to drive that far. I decided to risk it and, as I drove the car, I massaged both hands vigorously by rotating them on the steering wheel with a rather firm grip. Both the headache and the pain disappeared in a matter of minutes and did not return, allowing me to go about my business.

Mrs. L. C. P.

Stomach and Gall Bladder Relieved

Dear Mildred Carter:

I am studying this book *Healing Yourself with Foot Reflexology* and I just want to tell you how beneficial I am finding the instructions. Pains in the stomach and over the gall bladder were relieved almost at once.
Thank you.

Very truly,

M.F., Florida

Radiation Burns Treated with Reflexology

Dear Mrs. Carter,

A doctor told me to write to you and send for the reflexology book. He said that reflexology is akin to acupuncture and that all of this work was done by the ancient Egyptians.

My husband had his legs burned by radiation and clots keep forming, and we have to keep working them out. I use the reflex treatments every night on him and they help very much. They have also relieved the pain of sciatica, for which he is very thankful.

I am having wonderful results with reflexology and use it on all my friends who will let me. So grateful to you.

J.C., Texas

CHAPTER 31

Help Avoid
Female Discomforts
with Reflexology

Personal experience over the years has proven that reflexology helps the body relax, improves circulation, and alleviates problem conditions with the sex glands.

I suffered from my first period. Every month, I went through an agony of pain equal to labor pains, although I did not know this until I married and my first baby was born. The doctor was in a hurry to go home, so he took the baby with instruments and pulled my uterus loose from the muscles. This caused a constant feeling of discomfort in the lower region of my body from the navel down. Anyone having trouble in the reproductive organs knows the feeling; everything hurts! Two years later, I had another baby with no trouble, and a few months later, the doctor operated and tied my uterus back into place.

Not long after this, I started having cysts on the cervix and had to have them burned off every few months. I was not the only one who suffered in the ensuing years. I could not be a normal wife or mother because I always had a dull, heavy feeling from the waist down. I was nervous and irritable. I was lucky to have a kind and understanding husband.

After we moved to Idaho, I had a bad spell and went to a doctor there who hurt me on examining me. He told me that I had cancer and that he had to operate immediately. I knew this was not true as I had just been to my own doctor before leaving California.

HOW OLD-FASHIONED DOCTOR ENDS FEMALE TROUBLES

I then went to another old-time doctor. His office looked clean, but outdated. When I told him my problems of many years' standing, he was furious, not at me, but at doctors. He said, "There is no reason in the world why any woman should have female troubles. The reproductive organs are the easiest to heal in the whole body because nature set them up to reproduce. They respond to the simplest of treatment." He cauterized the cyst and gave me a prescription. "You take this tonic and you will never have any more trouble." I asked him if I could have another baby and he said I was too scarred by cysts to carry one if I ever did get pregnant. Well, I did get pregnant one month after taking the tonic, and nine months later had a perfect baby girl.

We went back to California in a few months and I went into a drugstore to have the prescription filled. The druggist said he would send on to the doctor in Idaho for it. I waited for weeks and he kept saying it hadn't come in yet. One day, I got mad and told him I wanted it, so he said, "Oh, yes, we got it, but it called for some old-fashioned ingredients. We don't use the 'L.P.' stuff anymore." I told him what I thought—that if they used it, there would be no more drugs to sell to suffering women, and no more operations for the doctors to perform. He just laughed.

Reflexology and Tonic End Operations

I got along fine for several years after my baby was born. One day, I had pains in the lower part of my body. I went to my doctor and he said, "Cysts again," and I had to be cauterized once more. I thought, "Oh, no, here we go again." Then I remembered that wonderful old-fashioned doctor in Idaho. I went to the drugstore and bought a bottle of the "old-fashioned" patent medicine ("Lydia Pinkham") and I have never had trouble again.

That was forty years ago, and I have never been to a doctor since for female troubles. Of course, I then learned the technique of reflexology and never had to worry anymore, but I still keep a bottle of the "L.P. tonic" on my shelf. I used it for my daughters through their adolescent years. Even today, if they mention troubles in the region of the reproductive organs, I tell them to work their reflexes and take some L.P. tonic.

I tell you this story to let you know the needlessness of suffering from any kind of female disorders. The reproductive organs will heal themselves when nature is given a chance.

HOW TO STOP PAINFUL MENSTRUATION

Pain with menstruation, heavy flow, missing periods, or premenstrual syndromes are all disorders caused by physical and emotional changes in the body. These monthly troubles are discouraging, but with the help of reflexology you can control painful hours of menstrual cramps like magic.

I have helped many women get back on a healthy monthly schedule, reduce their bloated feeling, and turn their negative mood swings into positive ones. Reflexology relaxes and soothes the body. It is nature's method of electrifying and reinforcing natural energies throughout your entire body and, when used correctly, will help flush out toxic fluids and regenerate healing stamina.

With reflexology you will no longer need the deadening influence of drugs. You can relieve pain from your back and thighs, as well as those terrible contractions in the uterus, by the simple method of holding pressure on the wrist area of your hand. (See Photo 36, below, and Photos 37 and 38 on page 227.) Hold the pressure firmly for three to fifteen minutes and then change pressure slightly to one side, and then to the other. Keep in mind that you are pressing the reflex areas that affect the sex organs and activating the healing forces of nature.

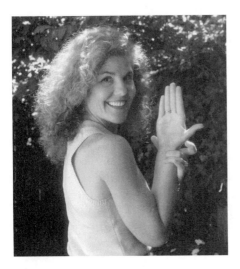

Photo 36: Position for working the reflexes to the lower abdomen.

Teens and adults with PMS have been able to help themselves with the use of reflexology. They simply work the reflex area to the ovaries, uterus, and to the endocrine system (see page 57) to regulate and balance these hormone-secreting glands. Each reflex is stimulated for only a few seconds at first; we do not want to overdo.

Helpful hand reflex methods:

- Press along zones one and two that correspond to the reflexes of your spine and its connecting muscles. Then slowly work the reflexes within the Magical V of each hand. (See Photo 58.)
- A press-and-pull movement along the edge of hands and wrists is very comforting. (See Illustration 4, page 22.)
- Work along the edges of all fingers to relax your nerves. (See Photos 5 and 6 on page 32.)
- Work the reflex points across the lower part of each hand, which is the reflex area to the lower abdominal area. (See Photo 36 on page 220.)
- To relieve headache pain brought on by menstrual distress, work around the thumbs.
- If you feel stressed, press and hold on the solar plexus points in the center of each hand to relax your nervous system. Once your spinal muscles, abdomen, and nerves relax, so will you.
- Using the Deluxe Hand & Foot Roller slowly between your hands (or slowly under each foot) will encourage relaxing circulation, which usually reduces the severity of menstrual difficulties and abdominal cramping.

Foot reflexology helps stop cramps: A technique of foot reflexology is especially helpful for relieving cramps. Simultaneously work the two reflex points that correspond with your ovaries and uterus. You will find these two points just below your inside and outside ankle. (See Photo 63, page 285.)

Use your thumb and index finger to squeeze and press this area on one foot for three minutes, and then repeat on the other foot to help balance your hormonal glands and stop cramps. It is best if you work the reflex points a week before your period is due to begin, and continue during the first three days of your period to combat menstrual difficulties.

A research report in *Obstetrics & Gynecology* is very exciting for those who suffer PMS. Terry Oleson and William Flocco conducted a clinical study to see if reflexology to the hands, ears, and feet actually helped reduce PMS distress. And the results were remarkable, as they showed a 46-percent reduction in PMS symptoms for women who had reflexology done to the correct reflex points, compared to only 19-percent reduction for those who received the placebo reflex pressure.

Special tips: Remember that calcium is one of the most important minerals of the body. Teens should have no less than 1,300 mg and adults need at least 1,000 mg of calcium each day. Some foods that contain calcium are milk, yogurt, cheese, and green leafy vegetables. Hormones that regulate calcium into your body will affect the level of pain, tension, and even your mood. Also helpful to stop cramps are manganese and Vitamins C and B_6. The old-fashioned herbal L.P. tonic helps relieve menstrual distress and cramping. You may want to check with your doctor before using any home remedy.

Nun Helps Sister Friend Back to Health with Reflexology

I think of you every day with gratitude. A little over a week ago a young Sister friend was feeling very ill and had gone to bed. "What's the trouble?" I asked "Your period?" "No," she replied, "I wish it were." She hadn't had one for a year. So I gave her a treatment and said I'd continue to do so for a month, then if nothing happened she should see a gynecologist. Next morning she could hardly wait to tell me it had already begun. And it continued normally.

So I am giving her a treatment every night and I am praying the cycle will be normalized. You can imagine my joy since you experience it constantly yourself.

I am feeling very well, perhaps thanks to one-half hour of massaging my feet every day.

With affection and prayerful wishes,

Sister L.M.

A word of caution: I want to sound a warning here to anyone who is pregnant. Do not use deep depression on the uterus or ovaries reflex. If these reflexes can start the menstrual period in just a few minutes, then it is quite conceivable they might also cause a miscarriage. However, I have used reflexology on many pregnant women, and not one of them ever had a miscarriage. In fact, every one of the mothers-to-be delivered beautiful healthy babies.

How to use Reflexology during Menopause

Menopause is nature's way of saying your childbearing years are over, but there are many wonderful, naturally healthy years to look forward to and enjoy. Reflex work to the points that correspond with the endocrine glands will help balance the hormonal activity of your body. You may notice the reflex areas of these glands are very sore to the touch during menopause. The pituitary gland continues to secrete sex hormones; however, after about forty years, the ovaries no longer respond to these hormones. The ovaries slow their production of estrogen (female hormone) and so menstrual periods become irregular and stop.

Work the sex gland reflexes as described in Chapter 32. Slowly work the reflex area to all endocrine glands, and up and down zones one, two, and three. Work the spinal and the urinary system reflex areas to relax menopausal difficulties. Work one hand and then repeat on the other hand.

Reflex help for hot flashes: Relaxation and reflexology are two of the best ways to treat hot flashes. Work the reflex areas to the reproductive glands around the wrists. At the same time do some slow deep breathing exercises and use meditation. Think of yourself swimming in a nice cool pool or taking a nice cool shower. Studies have shown that women who used this type of meditation and reflexology found that their body temperature did go down and their hot flashes were less frequent.

Remember to eat foods with high levels of phyto-estrogen, such as soybeans, tofu, alfalfa, barley, oats, apples, and pomegranates. In addition, Lydia Pinkham liquid is an herbal compound that quickly assimilates into the body, and will take away most symptoms of menopause distress and discomfort within a day, as it helps relieve stress in the area of the lower abdomen.

I have just given you the magic key with which to unlock the door that will free you from the pain and distress of being a woman, forever. All you have to do is use it. It is free!

Reflexology Stops Hot Flashes

Dear Mrs. Carter:

I want to tell you how much we have enjoyed your book on Reflexology, and how much good it has done. We have purchased about six books ourselves and given them away to members of our family and friends. Also we have told many of our friends about reflex therapy, and they have become interested and bought the book. I don't think there is anyone who it hasn't helped in one way or another.

As for myself, I began having hot flashes a few months ago and it stopped them completely. What a relief, the mysterious fainting spells also stopped.

My husband who is seventy years old was having trouble of some sort. We didn't know what. Doctors didn't seem to know either. One said he had diabetes, which it turned out he didn't have. Anyhow he was having spells where he would almost pass out several times a day. His back was pretty much out of line, which we didn't know. He had been going to a chiropractor for several years, but they couldn't seem to help much. So to make a long story short, he started with the foot reflexology. His passing-out spells stopped in about a week. He has worked on his feet for about a year now. He says he can feel the bones in his spine and neck move, and slip back and forth. He feels much better. So needless to say, he is a firm believer in reflexology.

Mrs. R.D.S.

CHAPTER 32

Using Reflexology to Treat Sex Glands

The reproductive organs are the strongest part of any species. I don't know of any part of the body that can cause more suffering and unhappiness over a long period of time than malfunctioning reproductive organs. When these organs are out of tune, then truly the whole system is rasping in disharmony.

THE IMPORTANCE OF SEX GLANDS

The reflexes of the gonads, or sex glands, in both male and female are of the utmost importance, not only in helping nature stimulate these reproductive organs and glands back to life if they are in a state of malfunction, but also to keep them in perfect order for the welfare of your whole system.

The testes of men and the ovaries of women are associated almost exclusively with their reproductive functions. While reproduction is unquestionably the most important function of the gonads, the hormones they produce have far-reaching effects on the body generally, and even upon mental activity.

Certain distinct cells of the ovaries and the testes devote themselves to the production of steroid hormones, while others evolve into spermatozoa and ova. Both functions are closely related to and controlled by the pituitary gland.

In Chart G on Endocrine Glands on page 57, you will see the position of the sex glands and organs, and you will see the position of the corresponding reflexes.

HOW TO ENHANCE THE HEALTH OF YOUR SEX GLANDS

In the wrist you will find reflexes to the ovaries, uterus, and fallopian tubes in the female; and the reflexes to the testicles, penis, and prostate gland in the male. Look at the Zone Chart on page 14 and notice how meridian line one runs down through the center of the penis, prostate, and uterus. You can see how the pituitary gland influences these organs in the center of the body, while the pinel, thyroid, and adrenals carry their influence to the ovaries and testes.

Since Mother Nature saw fit to move the reflexes of these most important glands from the bottom of the feet up to the ankles (probably so they would not become overstimulated as they were walked on), she may have moved the gonad (sex gland) reflexes to the wrists of the hands for a similar reason.

You can see how reflex stimulation around the wrists will affect the sex glands and organs involved, and help heal the whole lumbar area. To help invigorate these glands with the healing forces of nature, work not only the reflexes that directly correspond to the prostate, penis, or uterus, but also work the endocrine gland reflexes as well, since they are all interrelated.

Effective reflex procedures: With fingers under the wrist for support, place your right thumb on the inside left wrist, below the thumb. (See Photo 37.) Now, with a pressing, rolling motion, work this whole area, searching for a tender spot. When you find it, you will know you are on the right button. Keep working for a few minutes, then change hands, and work the reflex on the right wrist. Do not be surprised if you find one wrist more tender than the other, as this often happens.

By studying Chart D on page 13, we see that the thumbs of both hands should receive reflex work to stimulate the pituitary gland, which is in the center of the brain and is in control of hormones sent to the sex glands. Press the edge of one thumb into the center pad of the opposite thumb, giving it a deep rotating pressure to help activate the vital life force back into the hormone channels that are interconnected with the other sex glands.

How to help the prostate, penis, and uterus with reflexology: Congestion of the prostate gland, also the penis and uterus, can be helped by using reflexology on the entire lower lumbar area. You can see in Photo 37 how the thumb is placed on the inside wrist just below the thumb on the opposite hand. In Chart A, page 10, you can find the location of these organs. On Chart E, page 14, you will see how the zone lines run from fingers one and two down through this area to the toes. Also notice how they pass through the pituitary gland, which is located in the head.

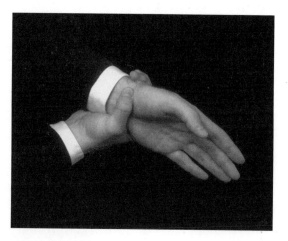

Photo 37: Position for working the reflexes to the prostate and penis on men and to the uterus on women.

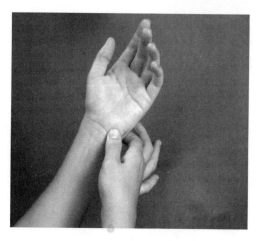

Photo 38: Position for working the reflexes to the ovaries on women and to the testes on men.

How to work the ovaries or testes: Now, let us turn to the reflexes for the ovaries in the female and testes in the male. Look at Photo 38 and see how the thumb is placed on the wrist on the same side as the little finger. Since the ovaries and testes are on each side of the body, work the reflexes in both hands. If there is a malfunction here, these reflex points will be tender. Concentrate on the side that is affected more.

The thyroid, adrenal, and other endocrine glands should be given special attention when there is trouble in this region of the body. Notice how many of these reflexes are crowded together in the center of each hand, so when one reflex is stimulated, the others also get their share. The Magic Reflexer will work well in activating the reflexes that correspond to these organs.

How to Lessen Pain with Reflexology

Remember, to stimulate and heal, we use an *agitating motion* in our reflex work. To quiet down or weaken pain, we use *pressure*. If you are trying to stop pain to the uterus, penis, or prostate, then it will be better for you to put pressure on the thumb. Use your fingers to search out tender spots on the thumb and, when you find them, hold a steady pressure for about 15 minutes at a time. If the pain occurs on one side, place pressure on the second or third finger on same side as the pain. You may need the help of reflex clamps to hold pressure on fingers for this length of time.

Hormonal Imbalances in Men and Women

Give yourself a "complete reflex workout" two or three times a week, giving special attention to each of your endocrine glands. When these precious control centers are not balanced, it will be trouble for a vibrant body. When there is a hormonal imbalance, it concerns every cell and tissue of the body. The imbalance can bring on pain, irritability, mental depression, muscle weakness, poor memory, swollen hands and feet, constipation, sexual dysfunction, and weight gain, just to name a few related problems. So put your mind at peace and facilitate your own healing, with the simple procedure of working all the reflexes to create harmony, and balance glandular activity within your whole system.

Malfunctioning Sex Glands

Both men and women who have suffered from malfunctioning sex glands know how the whole lower part of the body is affected. It feels as if infection has set in from the waist down, so let us work all of this lower lumbar area for relief. Reflex the entire wrist, working with a press-and-rotate movement clear across, from side to side and even up the forearm if it feels tender. (See Photo 54, page 282.)

Reflex Help for Prostate Problems

I have detected many troublesome prostate glands in men who came to me for other complaints. The congestion had not developed enough to cause any hostile symptoms, so the patients were not aware of the problem. I usually worked on their feet, which you can do also. However, if it is easier for you to reach your hands, you can renew circulation and help rebalance glands by just working along the insides of your hands and around the wrists. Either way, reflexology is an excellent treatment for correcting this condition when caught early.

Prostate troubles can affect men of any age, but it becomes more common after the age of fifty. If the prostate becomes enlarged, it can interfere with urine release. Some men must get up many times during the night to empty their bladder; others may experience a stinging sensation, which could be due to an infection.

Reflex points for the prostate are in the same location on each hand. Press the thumb of the opposite hand in the prostate reflex, in the fleshy part of wrist, on the thumb side of each hand. (See Photo 37 on page 227.)

Using a press-and-rotate movement, work reflexes to other organs that influence the health of your prostate, such as the liver reflex on your right hand. Also, work the entire reflex area to the urinary system, including the bladder, ureter, kidneys, and adrenal glands on both hands. Include a workout to the rectum reflex on the left hand, and work up and down the spinal reflex on both hands if there is pain in the lower back.

Look on Chart G (page 57) and notice where all the important endocrine gland reflex areas are located. Work each one of them to balance hormone stimulation. Rotate your wrists and ankles to keep the lymph moving, as a healthy immune system is very important to a healthy prostate.

How Prostate Is Cured Almost Immediately

Mr. A. reports: "I want to tell you how wonderful I think reflexology is. Although I am only in my early thirties, I have had prostate trouble along with other health problems for the past two years. After studying your reflexology hand charts, I decided to try it on myself. I worked all of the reflex areas in both wrists and felt almost immediate relief.

"Then I worked all of the reflexes in both hands. Now I am free of all prostate trouble and the rest of my illnesses seem to have vanished also. I feel great for the first time in two years.

"Thank you for introducing me to Reflexology. From now on it will have top priority in my family."

How a Doctor Cures Breast Tumor with Reflexology

Dr. Bowers told of a case of breast tumor, with two fairly good-sized nodes as large as horse chestnuts. The lady had made arrangements to be operated on by a prominent surgeon in Hartford. She postponed the operation for a few weeks on account of the holidays.

Meantime, she had been instructed to make pressure on the tongue and use rubber bands on the fingers for the relief of the breast pain, which he says brought quite complete relief. When she went to make arrangements for the operation, the surgeon found the growth so reduced in size that he was unwilling to operate. The tumor has since completely disappeared.

Dr. Bowers wrote, "This patient and the name of the surgeon who saw her before and after are at the disposal of any physician who may regard this as untrue."

How a Uterine Fibroid Disappeared

"A small uterine fibroid made a similar happy exit, as a result of pressure made on the tongue and the regular practice of squeezing the joints of the thumb and first and second fingers.

"Lymphatic enlargements, as painful glands in the neck, armpits, or groin, yield rapidly to this pressure. And while no claims are made to the effect that cancer can be cured by zone therapy, there are many cases in which pain has been completely relieved, and the patients freed from further use of opiates, and in a few cases the growths have also entirely disappeared."

(From the files of Dr. Bowers, who has since departed from us.)

CHAPTER 33

Reflex Techniques for Easier Childbirth

Any woman who has gone through the pangs of childbirth, with or without drugs, will welcome the news of a natural, less painful method of delivery. Any technique, no matter how improbable it sounds, is worthy of consideration by a physician, and especially the parents-to-be.

They need only to turn to nature and the use of modern "push button" approaches to bring their baby safely into the world, without danger to the health of the mother or to their unborn infant.

With the help of reflexology, a woman starting into labor can press the reflexes in her hands to help relax the cervical muscles, which promotes dilation. This makes the delivery easier for the mother and child, and gives them both a better chance for life with less danger of complications setting in. This natural method of helping the mother deliver more quickly should be a great boon to doctors and nurses, and especially to the delivering mother and her baby.

DOCTOR LECTURES ON CHILDBIRTH

In a lecture to physicians on "Easy Childbirth," Dr. White stated:

> Any method calculated to render labor less of an ordeal—particularly when the method can possibly do no harm—is worthy of trial. There is absolutely no danger to either mother or child in its employment, for in almost every case in which Zone therapy (reflexology), has been tried, labor has been accelerated three hours or more, instead of retarded.

HELPFUL REFLEXOLOGY TECHNIQUES
FOR EASIER LABOR

The following reflexology techniques for easing pain during labor are in no way a substitute for qualified medical care. Always make sure your doctor is accessible.

One technique is to press on the inside of the wrist, on the thumb side of the hand. Press and hold this reflex point, maintaining constant pressure for ten to fifteen minutes. If the hands become tired, relax them for a few minutes, and then continue the pressure. Another reflex point that will relax the abdomen is the Magical V. (See page 34.) At the same time, if it's possible, press the soles of your feet hard against a footboard, which should have a rough rather than a smooth surface.

Another method is for the patient to hold two reflex combs, one in each hand with the teeth facing upward. She should exert pressure across the tops of the second and third fingers, and at the end of each thumb. Do not use ordinary household combs for this, as they could break under pressure and injure the fingers. Reflex combs are specially designed for the purposes of hand reflexology.

Reflexology Used Instinctively by Women in Labor

This method of help in time of labor is merely an amplification of techniques that have always been used instinctively by women. The clenching of hands, the crushing grasp on the hands of the husband or support person, are nature's own methods of bringing relief from pain during labor.

They are inadequate, however, because the pressures are not maintained for a sufficient length of time, and because the means for making the pressure are not sufficiently "sharp enough" to dig into the reflex points. In other words, nature knows what should be done, but we need to assist in the process. Reflexology merely increases the effectiveness of an already existing method by improving on it.

Special Tips Make Delivery Easier

It is very important that a pregnant woman and her husband or support person take a preparation-for-labor course. You will both learn the proper breathing techniques to use during the labor, and other special tips to help ease pain and make delivery easier. One tip is to apply warm Vitamin E oil to the region between the anus and the genital organs to help keep skin soft and elastic, hopefully preventing an episiotomy. All my girls rubbed cocoa butter on their belly, hips, and breasts to help make skin supple and hydrated, which helped them avoid getting stretch marks.

You both might acquire new knowledge of reflexology, learning how it enhances circulation, as does a good back massage. Remember, renewed circulation helps the blood move along easier, which will be less stressful for the heart and other organs during delivery.

Use Reflex Comb Technique Only When Doctor Is Present

Before going on to some case histories, I want to emphasize most strongly to those readers who are expecting a baby, not to try this method by yourselves, or you might suddenly find yourself alone with a newborn baby! In these days of poor nutrition or indifference to proper diets, lack of enough exercise, etc., there could be complications, in which case you would need your doctor with you. It might mean the life of your baby or even your own, so be sure that the doctor is available.

I have never delivered a baby myself, but I wish I had known of this method when I had my own first baby delivered by instruments, and again when I was forced to have a Caesarean with a later child after hours of suffering.

Now I am going to give you some actual case histories taken from the files of prominent medical doctors who did use zone therapy (reflexology) when natural methods of healing and doctoring were still considered in style.

Young Mother Has Painless Delivery When Doctor Uses Reflexology

Dr. R.T.H. Nesbitt of Waukegan, Illinois gives this report on his first experience with zone pressure in a confinement case after attending a lecture by Dr. White:

"As I was expecting a confinement call every hour, I told Dr. White and he gave me some special pointers concerning this work. Last night I was called to attend what I expected would be my last case of confinement, as I have been doing this work so many years that I intended to retire. From my last night's experience, I feel as if I should like to start the practice of medicine all over again.

"The woman I delivered was a primipara (one who had never had a child before), and who, therefore, because of the rigidity of the bones and tissues, has a more difficult labor.

"When severe contractions began, and the mother was beginning to be very nervous and complained of pain, at which time I generally administer an anesthetic, I began to press on the soles of the feet with a big file as I could find nothing else. I pressed on the top of the foot with the hands where the toes join the foot. I exerted this pressure over each foot for about three minutes at a time. The mother told me that the pressure on the feet gave her no pain whatsoever.

"As she did not have any uterine pain, I was afraid there was no advancement. To my great surprise, when I examined her about 10 or 15 minutes later, I found the head within two inches of the outlet. I then waited about 15 minutes and found the head at the vulva.

"I then pressed again for about one or two minutes on each foot, the edge of the file being on the sole of the foot and my thumbs over the metatarsal-phalangeal joints as before. In this way I exerted pressure on the sole of the foot, and pressure on the dorsum (top) of the foot for about three minutes at a time, with my thumbs doing each foot separately for 1½ minutes. Within five or ten minutes the head was appearing, and I held it back to prevent tearing. It made steady progress, the head and shoulders coming out in a normal manner. Within three minutes the child—which 'weighed in' at 9½ pounds—was crying lustily. The mother told me she did not experience any pain whatever, and could not believe the child was born. She laughed and said, 'This is not so bad!'

"Another point that is very remarkable is that after the child was born, the woman did not experience the fatigue that is generally felt, and the child was more active than usual. I account for this on the principle that pain inhibits (prevents) progress of the birth, and tires the child. But as the pain was inhibited, the progress was more steady, and thus fatigue to both mother and child was avoided."

Reflexology Used to Shorten Labor

A Massachusetts doctor supplements the above case with several others, equally revolutionary. To insure brevity and accuracy I quote the doctor's own words:

Case 1. "Multipara (a woman who has had previous confinements), mother of four. Shortest previous labor eight hours. Had had a laceration of cervix (neck of womb) with her first child. Also one forceps delivery.

"When labor commenced she was given two aluminum combs to hold and instructed to make strong pressure upon them with the view of inhibiting pains. The combs were to be used especially on the thumb and first and second fingers. These combs were notched slightly and roughened on the ends so as to stimulate the side surfaces of the thumbs more effectively.

"Was called at four A.M., arrived at 5:05, and the baby had just been born. The patient reported that she had been in bed for only 15 minutes. There had been one severe pain—that was when the head delivered.

"There was no exhaustion following, as with previous labors, and she said laughingly, 'I believe I will be able to get up this afternoon, Doctor.'

"The afterbirth delivery seemed to be stimulated, and her pains controlled by gently stroking the back of her hands with the teeth of the combs. She became relaxed and drowsy from this stroking, and fell asleep and slept almost through the night, perfectly free from pain."

How Reflexology Caused an Unexpected Birth

A friend tells me the following story about her daughter's experience with reflexology:

"A few weeks before my daughter's baby was due, I told her about the reflex method to painless childbirth as I had learned from you. I explained how to press the hands and fingers with a comb or solid object to relax the tension of the uterus when it was time for delivery, but I forget to warn her not to use this method until she was sure that labor was starting and that her doctor was near.

"They lived out in the country, and her husband was working close to the house.

"This is what she told me. 'One afternoon as I lay on the couch to rest, I decided I would try the comb method you had told me about so that I would know how to do it when it was time for the baby. I got two ordinary combs, remembering that you had said they might break if one wasn't careful. I started pressing the teeth into my palms and then into my fingertips, just trying them out.

"'I felt so quiet and relaxed after a few minutes I guess I just kept doing it. Then suddenly something broke in me and there was water all over everything—then I knew the baby was coming. I felt one little pain and there it was! I didn't know what to do. I wrapped it up in my husband's coat laying close by, and walked out to where he was working. He nearly fainted as he saw me all bloody. He rushed us to the hospital, and we were both fine. The next time I have a baby, I will use the combs and reflexology, but I will be sure I am not alone, and that someone is right there with me.'"

If you want to use the reflexology method to help you have an easier delivery, remember the experience of the above young mother and don't try it until you are sure that it is time for the baby to be born—and don't be alone. Also read "A Word of Caution" on page 222.

HOW REFLEXOLOGY HELPS MOTHERS BREAST-FEED THEIR BABIES

While we are talking about the advantage of easier childbirth, let's take one more look at the advantage of birth without being over-medicated and consider the future of the baby. We all know that breast-feeding is the most natural and healthful way of nourishing babies from birth to weaning time. We know that a substance in the human mother's milk protects infants against many infectious diseases.

A British doctor announced recently that "breast-fed babies are not nearly so susceptible to heart attacks when they grow to maturity. And breast-fed infants are susceptible to far less digestive trouble than bottle-fed ones."

Doctors Niles Newton and Michael Newton—a husband and wife team of psychologist and obstetrician—have devoted years to studying every aspect of breast-feeding as it affects mental and physical health of the infants and mothers. They are strong in their feelings about the necessity of breast-feeding for good psychological and physical health.

There is no feeling in the world that can compare with the joy of holding your newborn baby close in your arms and feel his little mouth taking the nourishment from your body as nature intended.

How I Relieved Pains of Pregnant Woman

A neighbor girl came over to my house one afternoon and asked if I would drive her to the doctor. Her husband was at work and we were 20 miles from town. I asked her what her trouble was. She said she was pregnant and had terrible pains in her side. She was only three months' pregnant, and I felt she had better see her doctor so I drove her the 20 miles to his office. He could not find anything wrong with her and told her it was just one of those things she would have to put up with.

I talked to her about reflexology and learned she had taken the treatments several times from a friend of mine near where she had lived. When she got home, I gave her a treatment. On her next visit to the doctor, she told him how the reflex treatments helped her and he said to continue them.

All through her pregnancy the pain kept recurring at intervals, but the treatments stopped it for several days and sometimes for weeks. We never knew what had caused the pain which was located low down in her side. She had a very hard time with her first baby, developing a heart problem and having to have several specialists.

I took her to the hospital when it was time for the baby to be born. In view of the trouble she had with her last delivery, there was a heart specialist on standby.

She had the baby by Caesarean section with no complications whatsoever. We felt that the reflex treatments given during her pregnancy were responsible for the safe delivery of her baby, and for the fast, uncomplicated recovery and feeling of well-being in the following months.

How Reflexology Helped Mother-to-be Avoid Labor-inducing Drugs

Dear Ms. Carter:

I wanted to write to express my gratitude to you. Your books on hand, foot, and body reflexology have helped my family and me so much. I especially appreciate your advice on general health matters such as diet, the electrical energy surrounding the body, the importance of drinking water, and more.

I would like to share a story with you: I didn't go into labor on schedule after nine months of a normal pregnancy. The doctors gave me two more weeks, at the end of which they would admit me to the hospital and induce labor. I didn't want that to happen as I had planned for a natural childbirth and didn't want any drugs. The night before I was to be admitted to the hospital, I was still not in labor. I started to (gently) massage the arm/wrist reflexes to the uterus, thinking that either this would work or I would have to consent to the labor-inducing drugs the next morning. I fell asleep in bed as I massaged, and woke up at 3 in the morning with a "stomachache." That "stomachache" turned out to be the start of the labor process, and I delivered a normal, healthy boy the next afternoon without any drug interaction.

Not only have your books helped my health and that of my family, but also affirmed my own quiet belief that the natural way of life is truly the best way to live and to raise children.

Thank you so much for everything!

Jennifer P.

CHAPTER 34

Reflexology for Children

When given half a chance, all children have a natural instinct to turn to nature for food, health, and a happy way of life. This is why reflexology is becoming so popular with the younger generation; even very young, preschool children are able to give a treatment of reflexology to their parents and other members of the family. Many of these youngsters are quite fascinated by the sincere appreciation they get from a previously complaining relative.

Reflexology can be a continuous source of comfort, and it is always available to us no matter what our age. Note in Photo 39 how

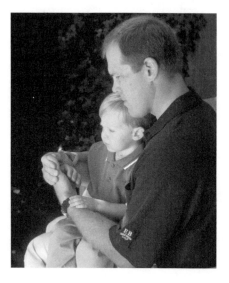

Photo 39: Teach children the safe and easy way to maintain perfect health with the natural use of reflexology.

239

intense the small boy is in learning where the reflex points are located in his dad's hands.

How to Maintain Your Child's Health

To maintain the body in perfect health as your child is growing, the endocrine system is of the most importance. If you feel that your child is not developing as he should, turn to the endocrine glands. If the child seems to be growing too fast, or not growing so fast as is considered normal at this age, your doctor should be consulted. Then turn to working the reflexes of the endocrine glands, especially the pituitary gland.

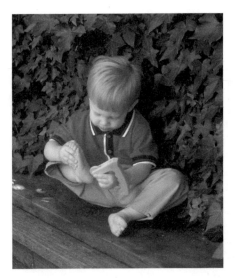

Photo 40: How a child's natural instinct helps him find nature's method of preserving good health.

Situated in the center of the head is the pituitary gland. It produces a number of hormones, including the growth hormone. When this gland is underactive, it produces a very small person; when overactive, it produces a giant. In the pad of both thumbs (and in the pads of the big toes) you will find the reflex point to the pituitary gland.

Reflexology does not alter genetic size, as it only helps balance hormonal secretions; it does not change the DNA. (Refer to Chapter 6 and learn the importance of the whole endocrine system.) See in Photo 40 how a child turns to reflexology in search of a natural way to improve health.

REFLEXOLOGY IS GOOD PREVENTION

There is a saying, "An ounce of prevention is worth a pound of cure." When it comes to our children's health, we will do whatever it takes to keep them safe, and prevent them from being sick or feeling pain.

Reflexology energizes the healing zones and helps promote a curative aspect to keep the body and mind functioning smoothly. It also stimulates lymph to help fight diseases and renews circulation to oxygenate blood for good general health.

Many doctors are now encouraging the use of reflexology since it is easy to do and can cause no harm when done as directed. First, teach your children to work the endocrine glands' reflexes. Once you teach them how to search for sore spots, nature will guide them to the right buttons and the correct pressure to use. You will be amazed at your child's natural instinct of turning to reflexology, especially when marvelous happenings occur through their search for a simple and better way to good health.

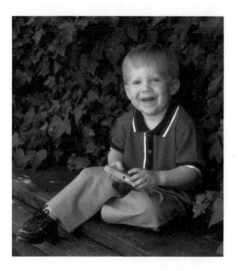

Photo 41: Two-year-old enjoys working the reflexes in his finger-tips.

Children Use Reflexology to Help Others

We can teach our children to use the benefits of reflexology, not only on themselves but also to help others overcome such complaints as muscle cramps or an upset stomach. They will enjoy helping their family and friends by showing them how to reflex thumbs and fingers, including the webbing between fingers to reduce nervous tension or headaches.

Both youth and seniors need compassion and healing in this day of high stress in our schools and in society. Reaching out a kind hand and using the healing methods of reflexology will benefit many who are discouraged or ill. Reflex therapy often relieves pain within minutes when there is a need. In addition, it can be used in cases of an emergenc to alleviate pain and quiet nerves until a doctor arrives.

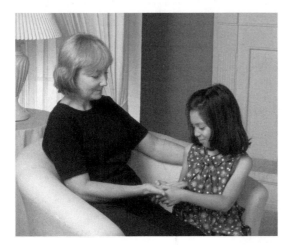

Photo 42: It is very rewarding for children to take an active part in helping others.

Teacher Uses Reflexology to Calm Nervous Tension

A teacher reports: "I want to tell you how reflexology has helped me in working with children, both in the schoolroom and out on the playground.

"Children of today seem to be under a high tension. It takes a lot of patience and calm nerves to cope with them. I used to be in a continued state of nervous tension, but since discovering reflexology, I can calmly handle any situation that arises.

"I 'keep my cool,' as the children say, by working the nerve reflexes in my fingers and thumbs inconspicuously even while I am teaching.

"I only wish I could teach the art of reflexology to the children. I am sure we would have healthier and happier children in the schools, and they would be better adjusted as adults in the future."

V.P, California

Children Use Reflexology in Sports

Many children who are involved in the field of sports are learning to rub the nerve reflex centers in their fingers to relieve tension just before going into competition, even inconspicuously during a game. Teens have learned that this quickly relaxes pent-up nerves, thus helping them to enter the game calm and cool. One young man is convinced it gives him a better chance of helping his team become the medal winners.

Reflex help for the weekend athlete: Whether you are fun loving or fearless, you must always have great balance and keep your body in good shape. Reflexology to all five zones on both hands will balance your *chi,* your vital energy. Further, work the reflex area at the base of your fingers to enhance eyesight and hearing, as they must be clear for peak performance.

When your muscles hurt: If it is a strain or a sprain, reflexology can help speed the healing process. Work the reflex to your liver and heart to promote fast recuperation and help increase your strength. In addition, do some deep breathing exercises to oxygenate muscles for a faster recovery and more power.

A helpful tip: Drink several glasses of water every day to promote healing. Stretch before and after all athletic adventures, to stay flexible. Use reflexology to improve your circulation and to energize your mind and body. Reflex all fingers to relax your nerves so that you will enjoy your sport and have fun.

Be a Winner with Reflexology

Reflexology will help you come out a winner every time if you will use it for any ailment or pain that might befall you. Don't leave this wonderful healing art for the younger generation to discover. Join them in their enthusiasm for nature's way to health through reflexology and you, too, will enjoy a fuller, happier way of life in perfect health for as long as you live.

Reflexology in Undeveloped Countries

Many of our younger people and our retired folks are going across the sea to bring light and comfort to those who are struggling in undeveloped countries. I hope that they will take the knowledge and understanding of reflexology with them, so that they may show others how an act of nature can help them regain their health.

I hope that reflexology will be used and taught whenever possible in their travels. They can share it with people who will use it to build a life of good health for themselves, their family, and their friends. It could be the foundation upon which to help free an entire country from suffering.

Reflexology, May God Bless You Forever!

Dear Mrs. Carter,

My grandchild, age five, had a sunstroke. I gave him reflexology for about ten minutes, took him to the hospital for further treatment, but there was no sign of brain damage—only a light fever. They kept him in the hospital for observation. The following day I went to the hospital and found him waiting to be taken home. The doctor asked me what method I used, as our boy told them that I pressed his hands, and that was why he felt so well. They could not believe my story. It is mind over matter, they said.

I told the doctor this method is "reflexology." Can you eat it, he asked. I said, if a person could eat reflexology there would not be one sick person on this earth. I told the doctor "a good full flow of water cannot run through a clogged pipe, the pipe must be cleaned of all obstructions to get the full flow of water through. This is true of your veins, the network of nerves, and also the invisible energy channels that promote renewed health." I also told him that reflexology is fifty years or more ahead of medication. Needless to say, he was not too happy with me. I can't blame him, as little does he know about this Godly method.

"Reflexology, may God bless you forever!" I am so indebted to you, Mrs. Carter, and the only way I can repay you is to continue helping myself and others with reflexology. I am a great believer in God and I know He was the one who led me to you. I am 63 years young, but I have changed the clock to 50 years, as I renewed magnetic energy for a fuller, happier, healthful life.

May God Bless you for your wonderful books.

Sincerely,

C. B., South Africa

Minister Encourages Boy Scouts to Use Reflexology

Dr. Edwin F. Bowers related that a minister, who taught his Boy Scouts "zone therapy" (reflexology) methods with special reference to curing themselves of coughs and other common ailments, found it effective. He stated further that the boys also found it valuable in their "First Aid to the Injured" work. One can readily understand that the analgesic effects of reflex pressure can be a factor in eliminating shock from pain whether in camp, at home, or a sudden onset of illness in the middle of the night when emergency help is not available.

To quote Dr. Bowers, "Zone Therapy opens up a tremendous field, so the more experiments we have, the sooner everyone will know just how tremendous and useful and marvelous it is."

CHAPTER 35

Glandular Disorders May Cause Alcoholism and Drug Addiction

"Can you help alcoholism?" is the cry of so many as they reach hopeless hands out of the darkness of despair.

Yes, reflexology can help those who are lost in the clutches of alcohol or drugs. These words should be like the tolling of a bell ringing out a new hope of freedom to thousands who suffer from these devastating diseases. There are few diseases that can bring as much distress into the lives of the victims and their families as drugs and alcoholism.

How Malfunctioning Adrenal Glands Are to Blame

In his book *The Encyclopedia of Common Diseases,* J.I. Rodale says:

> Alcoholism is a glandular disorder, and we can compare it with diabetes, as neither can properly metabolize carbohydrates. In the case of diabetics, not enough insulin is produced by the pancreatic gland which has this function, so the patient suffers from high blood sugar.
>
> In the case of alcoholics, there is too much insulin rather than too little, with the result that the alcoholic has low blood sugar. What causes the extra insulin that causes the low blood sugar? Apparently, the function of at least two glands is involved—the adrenals (it is the cortex or covering of these glands that is involved), and the pituitary which regulates the adrenals.

E.M. Abrahamson, M.D., in his book *Body Mind and Sugar,* says:

> Alcoholism is caused by a deficiency in the adrenal cortical hormones—those hormones whose action is antithetical to insulin.
>
> The trouble may not be in the adrenal cortical itself, however, but in the master gland, the pituitary, which for some reason fails to stimulate the adrenal cortical glands as it does in normal operation of the endocrine system. It is believed, moreover, that this disability of the pituitary is not caused by the alcoholism itself but antedates its development.
>
> Hyperinsulinism, with its chronic partial blood sugar starvation, is an essential underlying cause of alcoholism.

If what these experts say is true, then we know that by energizing the vital life force into the endocrine system with reflexology, we can help nature return these glands back into normal functioning, thus helping the person who is afflicted with alcoholism return to a normal life.

HOW TO HELP THE ALCOHOLIC WITH REFLEXOLOGY

After reading the above explanation regarding the cause of alcoholism, it is plain to see how important the endocrine glands are. So we must first concentrate on reflexes to the pituitary gland that sends chemical messengers, called *hormones*, through the blood to control the body's need for alcohol. Its reflex point is located in the center of the pad on each thumb.

Next we will move down to the adrenal reflexes in the hands, as shown in Photo 33, page 204. Stimulate this reflex in each hand with the press-and-rotate technique. You will probably find reflexes to these glands quite tender at first, so be gentle.

After working the reflexes just mentioned, you can move on to the other endocrine gland reflexes. (Refer to Chart G, page 57.) Be sure to give each of these reflexes your special attention, since we have learned that if one important hormone-producing gland is out of balance, it will throw all the others out of harmony. Remember, when this system is in perfect order, the whole body will soon be able to adjust back to normal functioning.

To improve circulation, work five minutes or longer on the reflex to the heart, which is a large area found on the left hand. In addition, work the reflex area to both lungs, found in the upper pads of each hand.

Continue your reflex work by stimulating reflexes that interact with the glands. Remember, the whole internal body must be in perfect balance. You will want to work the liver reflex on the right hand and then the kidney reflex on each hand. The liver and the kidneys work together, and one does not function properly without the other. Therefore, we must give them equal reflex stimulation.

Search for tender reflex areas and give them extra attention, encouraging renewed energy currents to help remove poisonous waste that may have formed in the liver. Reflexology helps improve circulation to flush out poison from the liver through the kidneys. The kidneys filter it from the blood and then dismiss it from the body with water as urine.

Alcoholism is a much-misunderstood disease: The key word is disease, which many do not understand. Wives and husbands nag, children weep, doctors scold, and the bars get richer. Through it all the agonized and helpless alcoholic suffers more shame, pain, and bewilderment than anyone else involved.

Reflexology gives new hope to the alcoholic: So let us not condemn, but hold out a helping hand and show them that the answer lies *in their own hands.* Just by working the reflexes to certain glands and organs, every person who is afflicted with the disease of alcoholism may return to a normal state, free of his or her craving for alcohol.

REFLEXOLOGY HELPFUL IN TREATMENT OF DRUG WITHDRAWAL

Just as there is new hope for the alcoholic, reflexology offers a way back for the drug addict.

It has been discovered that by inserting an electric needle in the lobe of the ear of a drug addict, he or she returns to normal without the pain of withdrawal symptoms.

Reflexology can be used to accomplish the same results, by holding a tight pressure on certain reflex points in the lobes of the ears for a period of five to ten minutes or more; then relax the pressure. Repeat this for as long as needed, or until the patient recovers and feels he or she has no more need of the treatment.

Patients can easily use this method on themselves by pressing each ear lobe between their thumb and forefinger, if one has the composure to hold this position for the length of time needed. If not, they could try self-help tools to exert pressure on the ear lobes. Clothespins might be too tight for this tender area. However, the Reflex Clamps can be used with ease, while sitting, in a prone position, or even while standing.

The Magic Reflexer can also be a big help when needed. Fold fingers around the reflexer and hold it up to the ear lobe. Hold the reflexer in the palm of the hand, press one of its "little fingers" in the front of the ear lobe; now place your thumb against the back of the ear lobe and press them together. This gives added strength for longer pressure.

One problem for those with an occasional hangover (or for anyone who encounters them) is the morning-after taste in the mouth and bad breath, which is very displeasing to say the least. It is because the tongue harbors plaque and bacteria after drinking alcohol. The best way to clean the mouth is by brushing teeth, flossing, and using the Stirling Tongue Wand to eliminate the cause of bad taste and that terrible breath odor. (Refer to Chapter 9 for more details, and see Photo 64 on page 286.)

Reflex therapy offers help to the person trying to regain his or her strength, whether from an occasional hangover or as an alcoholic. Each would like a quick and painless recovery. Reflexology can be helpful to all those who are trying to withdraw from the habit of drinking. It improves inner health by restoring glands and organs to normalcy, thus rebalancing the body so it will once more become a melody of beauty and balance, free of all abnormal cravings.

Two Out of Three Alcoholics Have Lost Desire to Drink

Dear Mildred Carter,

I already have purchased your *Hand Reflexology* and *Body Reflexology* books. You have been an inspiration to me. I have studied other books, and they have been okay. But your books have been so helpful, and your eagerness to share with others has encouraged me to help others.

CHAPTER 36

Reflexology for Those in Wheelchairs

I have heard from many grateful readers who praise the use of reflexology. Many say they are in wheelchairs and are unable to get much exercise. However, with the stimulation of pressing reflexes under the skin, they have noticed positive changes in their health.

Others are having a more difficult time. Nervousness and frustration seem to discourage those who wonder what to do when a part of their body is paralyzed, or extremities are missing due to amputation. I will answer this question by telling you first to look at the Zone Chart on page 14.

You will see how the meridian lines run down through the full length of the body, starting at the top of the head and ending in the fingers and toes. If you are not able to move your arm or leg, or if it is absent, the zone lines would still follow through to the point at the end of that arm or leg.

For amputees, the zone lines run through the body and end where the limb stops. The reflex points would be in the ending nerves. They would be congested, but still be there. It is important to remember the body is but a temporary house for our immortal soul, so discover who you *really* are inside, then you can create a bright and healthy future for yourself.

How Hand Reflexology Helped a Friend

I met Butler in front of a store several years ago. He was a very nice looking man in his 60s, sitting in a wheelchair. He had a great smile, and said his name was Butler, but "everyone calls me Buddy." We talked for awhile about the puppies his grandchildren were trying to give away, and then started talking about ourselves. I mentioned reflexology, and asked if he had heard of it. He had read something about foot reflexology, and wondered how he was supposed to use it since he had very little feeling in his feet.

We talked about working other reflex areas, such as in his hands and his body, like the ears, and tongue, which all work to good advantage. I explained the remarkable benefits of working the reflexes in his hands. Hands are so convenient and can be easily reflexed while in a wheelchair or in bed. Reflexology is suitable for people to use anywhere, and can be effective anytime of the day or night. I happened to have an extra Deluxe Hand & Foot Roller in my car, and asked him if he would like to try it.

Less than a month later, I received a call from Buddy; he told me that he had worked his fingers and hands daily with the reflex roller. To his surprise, he felt it worked like a miracle, and stopped pain from many sources. Reflexology definitely made him feel better. It gave him unexpected energy that he never had before. He had no idea what the tender reflexes were stimulating, and said, "Who cares, as long as it works."

Buddy was excited to tell me that one of the local nurses had taken an interest in reflex therapy and is working out a reflexology system for amputees and those who spend a lot of time in their wheelchairs. He added, "We are forever grateful. Reflexology is such a blessing to so many people!"

A Few Basic Reflex Procedures

Place your right thumb in the palm of your left hand, and wrap your fingers around the back of the hand. (See Photo 30 on page 185.) Use your thumb and fingers to press into the reflexes on both sides of the hand. This will feel as though you are trying to pinch your thumb and fingers together, right through your hand. Move your thumb in slow, small pressing circles.

Work the reflex buttons in thumbs and each finger, giving special attention to every joint and the webbing between all fingers. Work the back and front of your whole hand, and include working around the wrist and forearm.

Using the Referral System

If a hand is crippled or missing, work the foot on the same side of the body. If a foot is crippled or missing, work the hand on the same side of the body. Your whole body will benefit from the stimulation, whether the reflex is activated through the hands or the feet. Working the referral area to the corresponding energy zone will enhance recovery of a swollen or sensitive area on the *same side* of the body.

Self-Help Tools Benefit Circulation

Amazing reflex techniques have been used by many to help themselves renew healing circulation. It may be hard for you to reach the reflex areas, but with self-help tools, you will find it's easy to work on your own hands or feet. Working the reflex points helps flush toxins from the body to ease swelling and inflammation that cause pain. Try reflexology; it will make a powerful, positive difference in your health and happiness.

If extremities feel weak or are numb, you may need to press a little deeper to get good results. However, do not press too hard, as you might bruise the skin. The hand-held Magic Reflexer might work well for you. (See Photo 9, page 40.) Alternatively, the eraser on a pencil might also be very useful.

Most reflex areas do not require deep pressure to release the body's vital life energy. Nevertheless, tender reflexes do need extra attention, and although pressing hard is sometimes uncomfortable, chronically tense and sore reflex buttons need to be worked today, so that tomorrow or next week, the pain will no longer be there. So motivate your energy pathways and automatically boost your body's natural well-being.

Using the Deluxe Hand & Foot Roller on your hands can be very effective. Place the roller between your hands. Simultaneously push one hand forward and pull one back (see Photo 32 on page 196). Another method is to place the roller on a table, and with your palm on the "roller-fingers," press down and move it back and forth. (See Photo 43, page 254.)

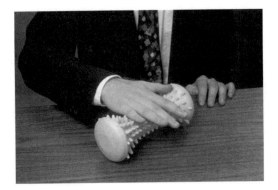

Photo 43: Place the roller on a counter, or the table, and roll it under one hand at a time to motivate circulation and renew internal energy.

Using the roller on your hand or rolling it under your feet will help stimulate energy currents throughout the body. It is beneficial for renewing circulation of lymph and blood to comfort the body and help it heal.

Do some foot reflexology: Use the roller to stimulate the reflexes in your feet. It is a very effective self-help item that can be used if you cannot comfortably reach your feet. Just place your deluxe roller on the floor and put one foot on it. First push your foot forward and then pull it back toward you. Repeat several times. The little "roller-fingers" will do the reflex work for you, encouraging rousing stimulation and promising renewed circulation. (See Photo 46, page 261.)

By experimenting a little, whether it is holding a steady pressure or using a gentle rotating motion on tender reflexes, you will find the technique that works best for you. It may take a little probing to find the secret reflex buttons hidden under the skin, but it can be done, and with very rewarding results.

HELPFUL TIPS

Your body needs exercise! Motion is very beneficial for your total wellness. So, move your arms and legs as much as you can. Bend your backbone from side to side, bend forward, and sit straight with your shoulders back. Lift your shoulders up to your ears, one at a time, then lift them both together. Pull in your stomach muscles; hold for a few seconds, and then relax. Repeat often to strengthen your abdominal muscles.

Deep breathing exercises: Widen your ribs and take in fresh air to oxygenate your blood. Cells will transfer oxygen through your bloodstream to help repair damaged tissues and assist the body in healing itself.

If you cannot get out of bed, you can consciously open up your ribs by mentally widening them. Think of your lower ribs expanding as you take in a deep breath. This is a wonderful exercise for your diaphragm, lungs, and heart, so do it often. Deep breathing is one of the most important things you can do for your health. See lung exercises on page 88.

Exercise all the muscles you can: For example, tighten your jaws and do some neck and eye exercises. (See Chapter 7 for eye exercises.) Continue to use reflexology; it takes commitment and hard work, but you will be rewarded with better health, as so many others are finding out.

One young man told me that obtaining reflex knowledge has given him a new outlook on life. He buys and sends our reflexology books to his family and friends in other states. He shares reflex techniques at the YMCA and with his church group. Reflexology keeps him actively involved with family, friends, and the public. He loves it!

Reflexology Helps Renew Interest in Life

Dear Mrs. Carter,

I can't begin to tell you what a change reflexology has made in my life. After losing an arm and a leg in an accident, I couldn't face living anymore. I was thirty-two and healthy when the accident happened. Afterwards, I just fell to pieces. I appreciate our conversation on the phone. I did take another look at myself and decided that I would see this lesson in life through, and learn from it as I am supposed to. I sure don't want to come back and live it over again.

I first started by feeling for reflexes at the end of my leg. I was surprised to find so many tender spots. I worked the reflex areas on my hand, too, and was more surprised at the change I felt. I started to enjoy the feeling of massaging myself. I have found that I do not hate myself anymore. I can face who I am and realize that my leg and arm are still with me, only invisible to others.

I am now spending my time passing the word to other amputees as you told me to do. I have lots of energy and a happy interest in life, which I have not had for a long time. I owe it all to you, you are wonderful!

God Bless You Forever,

James B.R.

CHAPTER 37

Relaxing
Nervous Tension
with Reflexology

Why do some people clench their teeth and double their hands into fists when they are upset or under emotional stress? When suffering great physical pain, when angry or apprehensive, sometimes they sink their teeth into their lips, often hard enough to cause bleeding.

People perform these and many other natural acts because they are instinctive and scientific, and because nature knows her business. We do them involuntarily and automatically because they relieve pain and nervous tension, and produce a form of anesthesia.

Let us learn to use this release of tension by voluntarily using pressure on the reflexes, as in Photos 17 (page 109), 44 (below), and 47 (page 268). You will remember in Chart B (page 11) how all of the fingers are marked "nerves," so you should work the fingers to stimulate the nerves, or use pressure on them to calm nervous tension.

If you are one of those people who live under nervous tension and anxiety, then you had better turn to nature's healing forces of reflexology. This way you will learn what it is like to live in peace and harmony although there is strife and chaos all around you.

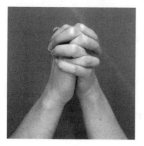

Photo 44: Position for relieving nervous tension by clasping the hands together.

Quickest Way to Calm Nerves

The quickest, yet most inconspicuous method of calming the nerves is to clasp your hands together, as shown in Photo 44, and squeeze tightly. By looking at Chart B (page 11), you can see how the act of pressing on all these nerve reflexes in the fingers at once must send a relaxing current into the whole system.

While you have your hands clasped in this position, work the fingers back and forth; move all the fingers to above the second joint and press-and-roll them together again. (See Photo 47, page 268.) Both of these reflex exercises work quickly to reduce nervous tension.

You may also want to refer back to Photo 17 (page 109). You will see how the tips of all fingers are placed against each other. When doing this exercise, press as hard as you can and hold for a few minutes. You may also use the reflex comb to press-and-hold on the ends of your fingers. (See Photo 61, page 285.) By the time you finish this reflex procedure, you may wonder where all the nervous tension has gone.

How Reflexology Helped Writer's Cramp

Dr. White tells of a case of neurosis—a writer's cramp—accompanying a neurasthenic condition. "This lady—unusually alert and intelligent—was a physical wreck. Sleepless, harassed by nerves in their most aggravated form, she was unable to hold a pen or to write more than a few minutes at a time until, on account of the pain and twitching of the arm, wrist, and fingers, she was forced to desist. She was also partly deaf from middle ear trouble.

"Several months' treatment, using the aluminum comb across the front and back of hands, and fingertips, and daily employment of the tongue depressor (or probe) for four or five minutes, brought forth a complete change in the patient's condition.

"It relaxed the terrible nervous tension—which was particularly marked along the course of the spine—enabling her to sleep at night and awake thoroughly refreshed in the morning. The writer's cramp was completely cleared up. A number of other conditions were also corrected, and her hearing was improved by fifty percent.

"This lady has since resumed her occupation as a private secretary—a position she was forced by ill health to relinquish more than two years ago—and now writes for hours at a stretch without any return of the cramp in the hand and the arm."

How Reflexology Cures Neuralgia in Tongue

My mother had what the doctors called neuralgia in a nerve in her tongue. I have seen her tongue double back into her mouth in a spasm and she would scream with pain.

She went to many doctors who gave her opiates (a medicine that contains opium or one of its derivatives to quiet the nerve and alleviate pain), not knowing of any other method of helping her. Finally, one doctor took her to a hospital in San Francisco and operated on her brain. He didn't help the nerve in her tongue, but cut a nerve to her throat which caused her to have severe choking spells. She had injections of Novocain™ in a nerve in her face which did help for a while.

Soon after I started to study reflexology, she came to visit me, and at the suggestion of my teacher, I searched out a very tender place in her toe and massaged it. After the first few minutes of reflex work, the pain in her tongue stopped and never returned. Of course, I kept working this reflex as long as she was with me and I taught her how to continue massaging her toe after she went home. She never had a recurrence of the terrible pain which caused her so much agony and trouble in the past.

How a Doctor Cured Tri-Facial Neuralgia

Dr. Roemer gives this report of a tri-facial neuralgia patient being permanently relieved by his application of reflex pressure.

He tells of a man who came to him who had been suffering from tri-facial neuralgia for more than two years.

"The patient had been advised to have the nerve cut. He had been unable to speak or eat for five days because of the severe pain that radiated over the entire left side of the face extending to the lower jaw the upper jaw, and up into the left eye. The pain was of a sharp piercing nature." He goes on to tell us, "I applied rubber bands on the joint of the thumb and forefinger (which would be No. 2) of the left hand, and in less than ten minutes he was talking and laughing. Nothing was said to him about the pain or what the rubber bands were applied for. I told him to apply them every half hour if the pain continued, and as the pain grew less, to lengthen the interval of application. He continues to use the rubber bands once a day, 'so I won't get out of the habit and to make sure the pain does not return.' He is now enjoying life better than he has for years."

HOW REFLEXOLOGY STOPS NERVOUS ANXIETY

If you are among the millions who suffer from anxiety, you will want to learn the helpful reflex approach that will naturally calm you.

How a doctor stops hand tremors: Dr. White tells about a case of a young man suffering from hand tremors, insomnia, and nervous exhaustion. "He had his fingertips clamped daily for one week, then for an additional three times more, at intervals of three days. After the eighth treatment, he had no further trouble with the tremors, slept like a baby, and was apparently relieved of all nervous symptoms."

If you want to stop hand tremors, try putting reflex clamps on all fingers for fifteen minutes daily or more often, for one week, and see what happens.

Clenching teeth relaxes nervous tension: If you are extremely nervous, there is a natural method of producing a soothing degree of relaxation. It is to clench your teeth (if you have a good set) and your hands for one minute at a time. Relax, and then tighten teeth and hands again, repeating several times. Repeat this exercise three or four times daily. You will find this method most helpful in overcoming nervous conditions.

HOW TO USE YOUR HANDS
AND FEET TO REDUCE STRESS

Stress affects the whole body in various negative ways, such as increasing blood pressure, nervous exhaustion, headache, excessive hunger, indigestion, diarrhea, sleeplessness, impotence, ulcers, and hair loss. You can see how important it is to sensibly relieve stress. Here are a few suggestions.

Work the pituitary reflex: Work on each thumb pad, and then work the pads of all other fingers. This stimulation will encourage healing energy to clear your brain and help you mentally release distress and tension.

Press into the center of your hands: A network of nerves is in the solar plexus area of your stomach. You will find this reflex in the center of each hand. It is marked with a star on Chart B, page 11. Press and hold this point while you do some slow breathing. Inhale as you count to seven, and exhale as you count to eight. Pressing this point on both hands will help you relax.

One technique of conveniently working the solar plexus and stomach area is to interlace your fingers. This opens up the hand for more effective reflex work. (See Photo 45.)

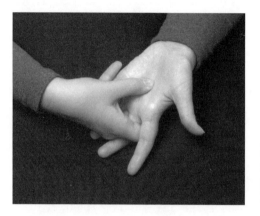

Photo 45: Position for applying pressure to the solar plexus point. This reflex is located in each hand.

Here is a great way to relax: When feeling stressful, some people like to do physical movements such as walk, swim, golf, or play basketball. Some people like to do relaxing hobbies, and others need to just lie down and rest. A wonderful self-help reflexology tool will make it easy for you to relax; it is enjoyable and beneficial to use.

First get into your most comfortable chair and do some slow, deep breathing. Next, place the Deluxe Hand & Foot Roller between your hands, or under one foot at a time, and roll it back and forth. If you have a rocking chair to sit in while doing this reflex technique, you will double the relaxing benefits. Do this exercise slowly for about twenty minutes or until you feel the stress and tension fade away from your whole body.

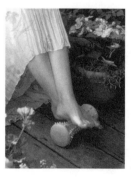

Photo 46: Roll the Deluxe Hand & Foot Roller slowly under one foot. For added pressure, place other foot on top; the roller's "little massaging fingers" will reward you with their magical relaxing benefits.

Reflexology Help for Claustrophobia

If you have ever been in a tight spot or an area with a small opening, you may have felt trapped and become temporarily claustrophobic. Some people get a pounding heart or dizzy feeling just from being in a room with other people. I knew one man who said he lost his balance every time he was on a moving elevator. Certain people faint and others even have seizures from intense fear. This is no laughing matter.

If you ever feel trapped or weak from fear, remove yourself from the area as soon as possible. Think of a happy place where you would rather be and slow your breathing.

Help yourself with reflexology: Place your fingertips together and press, slowly inhaling through your nose for seven seconds, and then relax your fingers as you slowly exhale through your mouth for eight seconds or more. Other methods are to overlap fingers so they touch between joints, or at the base of all fingers, and squeeze together. (Refer to Photos 17 (page 109), 44 (page 257), and 47 (page 268).)

If for some reason this exercise does not calm you, try pressing the solar plexus reflex point in the center of each hand. (See Photo 45 on page 261.) Once you calm your nerves, mentally assure yourself that you are okay. Do not drive until you are confident that you are completely in control of your emotions and over the symptoms of fear.

Reflexology Helps Alleviate Precarious Situations

A doctor told me that when body energy is low and contaminated with intoxicating beverage or narcotics, reflexology could be an ingenious plan. He sent me information on how to use reflexology to rid the body of unwanted spirit possessions. It is believed by many that an entity from another dimension can take possession of a body, especially where the vibrations (or energy) of the aura are lowered by alcohol or drugs.

How Doctor Uses Reflexology to Evict Possessions

Dr. Brandt told me that when a person is possessed by an entity, he or she usually has overactive adrenal glands. He says,

"The pancreas, adrenal, pituitary, and the pineal are all doubly active, but by using reflexology to return these glands to normal, active functioning, it doesn't leave any room for the extra spirit in possession and he either starves or leaves."

This information should give those who are working with serious mental cases something to think about. The Bible tells of people being possessed, and in many cases today there is suspicion that certain individuals may be possessed; but not many will come out in the open and talk about it. I hope that the simple technique of using reflexology on the endocrine glands will be tested by our doctors and psychiatrists in some of our sanitariums for the mentally ill.

For the success that I have had with these poor, confused people, I can only imagine the change that would take place in our institutions if the simple and harmless methods of reflexology were used for a few weeks.

Forceful life pulsations are manifested in the regions of the mind when these glands are activated with reflex stimulation, which also brings help for many types of mental depression.

Reflex Help for Mental Tension

Poor circulation causes mental tension. Low blood pressure and loss of oxygen to the brain will cause senility and lack of judgment. Work all reflex areas on the hands and arms, and work up and down each finger and thumb to relax mental anxiety. Work the tips and top pads of both thumbs and all fingers to improve blood circulation to the brain. In addition, rub hands together as if you are using invisible soap to wash them. This will help relax distress and worry.

I brought my 86-year-old mother back to normal with the use of reflexology after she became senile from the lack of oxygen after an operation. I know it works!

A helpful tip for mental confusion: The reason for mental confusion could be that your brain is not receiving its essential supply of blood and oxygen. To give it help, lie across your bed with your head over one side a little lower than the rest of your body. You can lie on your back or your abdomen. In this position oxygenated blood can easily flow to the head and nourish the brain. Soon cerebral tension will relax and cloudy thinking will become crystal-clear.

Using Reflexology to Cure Insomnia

If you are suffering from insomnia, try the following exercises. After you are comfortably settled into bed, interlock the fingers and clasp your hands together, as shown in Photo 44 (page 257), or press the finger tips firmly together, as shown in Photo 17 (page 109). Hold this position for ten to fifteen minutes, if you have not already fallen asleep by that time.

Yawn and stretch to relax: Another one of nature's relaxing exercises is to yawn and stretch periodically. This procedure stimulates a healthy action of the sympathetic nerves in all the zones, and cannot fail to be of great benefit.

REFLEXOLOGY IS IMPORTANT TO OUR HEALTH

The most important thing for our health is to learn how to relax. Anything that will teach us to relax without drugs and sleeping pills will prove to be a boon to humanity. For this reason, I am certain that the principle of reflexology will be a familiar and universally applied technique within the very near future.

How to Rebuild New Cells with Reflexology

The famous Canadian doctor, Hans Selye (*The Stress of Life*), said, "Life, the biological chain that holds our parts together, is only as strong as its weakest vital link."

You are as young or as old as your smallest vital links—the cells. The aging begins when your normal process of cell regeneration and rebuilding slows down. This slowdown is caused mainly by the accumulation of waste products in the tissues, which interferes with the nourishment of the cells. Each living cell is a complete living entity with its own metabolism. It needs a constant supply of oxygen and sufficient nourishment.

HOW HEALTHY CELLS STOP PROCESS OF AGING

When our cells are deprived of fresh air, sufficient exercise, and proper nourishment, they start to degenerate and break down. The normal process of cell replacement and rebuilding slows down and your body starts to grow old, in most cases before its time. Its resistance to disease will diminish and various ills will start to appear.

It is understandable that all of our glands, our bones, our skin, etc., are made up of these cells, so we must look first to the health of our cells.

Only about half of your cells are in the peak of development, vitality, and working condition. One-fourth are usually in the process of development and growth, and the other three-fourths are in the process of dying and replacement. The healthy vital life processes and perpetual youth are maintained when there is perfect balance in this process of cell breakdown and replacement.

If the cells are dying at a faster rate than the new cells are built, the process of aging will begin to set in. It is of vital importance that the dying cells are decomposed and eliminated from the system as efficiently as possible. Quick and effective elimination of dead cells stimulates the building and growth of new cells.

Here is where reflexology comes in as the most effective way to restore your health and rejuvenate your body by the simple process of stimulating the reflexes.

HOW TO ELIMINATE TOXIC WASTES WITH REFLEXOLOGY

When you work the reflexes, you are sending a vital life force through the entire system and reactivating organs and glands back to normal functioning. You are helping to clear out sluggish metabolism and constipation, and the consequent inefficient elimination that causes retention and accumulation of toxic wastes in tissues which interfere with the nourishment of cells, thus causing disease and premature aging.

How to replace old cells for new: Through this process of stimulating the eliminative glands with reflexology, you will be eliminating toxic waste products from your body. This will effectively stop the interference with nourishment of the cells, and soon the normal metabolic rate and cell oxygenation will be restored. Thus, you are on your way to replacing old cells for new! New cells mean new tissue, and a new, rejuvenated body.

THE IMPORTANCE OF OUR ELIMINATION ORGANS

You start this process of rebuilding healthy new cells by first increasing the eliminative and cleansing capacity of the organs that discharge wastes, which are the intestines, lungs, liver, kidneys, bladder, and the skin. When stimulation and pressure on the corresponding reflexes in the hands reactivate these organs, masses of accumulated metabolic wastes and toxins are quickly expelled.

This is why we tell you to work the reflexes for only a short time the first week or two. Do not work them more than every other day the first week. When these organs start throwing off poisons, the concentration of toxins in the urine can be many times higher than normal. These eliminative organs begin to concentrate on the cleansing of old, accumulated uric acids, wastes, and toxins from the tissues.

HOW TO START THE PROCESS OF REJUVENATION

To start the process of rejuvenation, you will give special attention to pressing and working the reflex to the liver. If you find tenderness in this area, you will know the liver is sluggish and lacks proper circulation. Use a firm pressure as you criss-cross the large reflex area across the right hand. Do not neglect to work the webbing between thumb and first finger. See Photo 7 on page 33.

Expel toxins by working the kidney and lung reflexes: Next, we will go to the reflexes of the kidneys, which are located in each hand. If you are not sure of the location, refer to Chart B (page 11). Notice how the thumb is pressed into the kidney reflex in Photo 33 (page 204). Work this a few seconds on each hand and then move up to the reflexes of the lungs, which are located on the pads under the fingers. Check the chart for this if the position is not familiar to you. Activate these reflex areas on both hands.

Revitalizing Skin and Bones with Reflexology

Now we come to the skin, which is the largest part of our eliminative system since it covers our whole body surface.

You will note in Photo 44 (page 257) how the hands are clasped, and in Photo 47 (page 268), notice how the fingers are pressed together. This is a natural stimulation to the whole nervous system.

By slightly squeezing and releasing the fingers several times, you will be sending a flow of the vital life force through the whole body, including the skin and the bones.

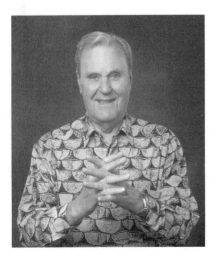

Photo 47: Squeeze base of fingers together, then squeeze at middle joints as shown here, to relieve distress and tension from numerous body systems.

Stimulating all the important elimination reflexes: This is where the Magic Reflexer is of great benefit. It seems to stimulate all of these important elimination reflexes simultaneously, and does a better job than just working one reflex at a time. When using the Magic Reflexer, be careful and do not over-massage the first time. This will not be easy to do . . . many people find it so stimulating they do not want to quit using it. So for the first week do not use the reflexer over two or three minutes at a time in each hand, no matter how good it feels.

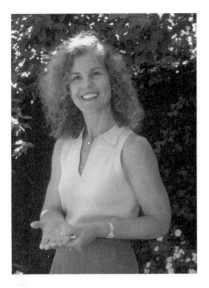

Photo 48: Reflexology promotes balance and normalization, bringing all systems into harmony and a state of good health, naturally.

BALANCING BODY CHEMISTRY
TO HELP CURE DISEASES

Alan H. Nittler, M.D., in his book *New Breed of Doctor*, tells us, "It is 'tissue weakness' that opens the door to one new disease after another, and no drug can build tissue strength."

Disease is an abnormal condition of the cells and tissue caused by an abnormal balance of body chemistry. In this abnormal condition is the only place abnormal cells can live and grow. When there is a balance of body chemistry, then normal cells are formed in which diseased cells cannot live, and healthy tissue is able to grow.

If we regulate the glands into producing their normal secretion to balance the body chemistry, we are giving nature a chance to build perfect cells, thus making the environment unfavorable to the diseased cells.

Regulating body chemistry: In reflexology, we know that by stimulating certain reflexes, we can regulate the balance of body chemistry by working the reflexes to all of the endocrine glands and organs. Whether the cause is from overstimulation or understimulation, reflexology will bring them back to a normal balance by sending the vital energy of life force into malfunctioning areas, thus regulating the chemistry of the body and giving nature a chance again to form normal cells in which the abnormal cells are no longer able to form.

I am not advising anyone to depend exclusively on any single remedy for a disease, but I do feel that what unnatural forces have disrupted, the healing forces of nature surely can put back into perfect working order.

In the book *Edgar Cayce on Healing* by Mary Ellen Carter and William A. McGary, M.D., there was some question of certain applications recommended by the great seer Edgar Cayce in many of his some 6,000 readings on healing. Edgar Cayce recommended Homeopathy (which is likened to Naturopathy, Osteopathy, and Chiropractic) as his choice of therapy. Remember that these recommendations came from a source that was not understood at that time and is just now being sought by those who are seriously seeking the answer to all diseases.

Edgar Cayce on the Aura

Here are some of the questions asked by the authors of *Edgar Cayce on Healing:* Is there an energy in the human body that we have not yet discovered? Is there an energy field around the body? Is this what has been called the aura?

Cayce described such a flow of energy in the form of a figure crossing at the area of the solar plexus. He also described the aura of the human as being a type of force field visible only to a few.

The practice of stimulating this energy life force to bring about therapeutic results has been used down through the ages, from the time of ancient Egypt.

MANY COUNTRIES USE METHODS RELATED TO REFLEXOLOGY

Many countries use related methods of what we call reflexology to achieve healing of all types of diseases.

We know of the Chinese and their acupuncture, using the needle method; then there is the Ju-Jube of Africa, where they use quills dipped in herbs that are applied under and around the arms and armpits to tap these life currents.

Japanese have their method called Shiatsu, in which they use the fingers as in our western method of reflexology.

India also has its special method of using this ancient therapy to heal the body by stimulating the flow of the energy field. Many other countries have been using therapeutic methods related to reflexology down through the ages.

Do you know that in recent years Russian scientists have photographed energies spurting out of specific reflex areas? That they have also photographed the aura; and that we are now able to do the same in this country?

These forces created by the human body are real and active. They are, in fact, observable and recordable in all living things.

Reflex therapy not only acts on the muscular structures of the body but also performs therapeutic duty to the uncoordinated functional organism. By using reflexology to all of the glands and organs, we balance the body so that its energies may be utilized in all its parts in restoration and regeneration of body tissues.

Cayce says that imbalance brings about certain glandular changes, particularly in the thyroid, which in turn disturbs the distribution of these energies or forces to their proper channels.

Cayce constantly talked of using the vibrations of several metals for healing, especially copper and iron to help activate the electrical energy forces.

In her "Special Financial Forecast," Marguerite Carter, the great Unitology Forecaster, tells us, "I believe with all my heart that we are on the threshold of the cure of diseases that are now taking so many lives, but the answer will not be 'new.' It is apt to be surprisingly simple and come about through a 'new way' of using something that has been at hand all along."

Many of us have sadly known of this forbidden secret for many years. But now, hopefully, under the pressure and demand of the masses, the growing conscious and humanitarian feelings of many doctors, and a benevolent God, perhaps we are at last approaching the end to untold suffering and fear from so-called incurable diseases.

I will not tell you how to work any certain reflex here, as I feel that you must concentrate on stimulating the reflexes to all of the organs and glands—especially endocrine glands—to achieve beneficial results. Study Chapter 6 on the endocrine glands and Chart G (page 57). Work the reflexes as directed to help nature overcome illnesses of all kinds. It costs nothing and can do no harm, so at least try it.

I am constantly in search of new methods of natural healing, and when I find one that is better than the positive and simple methods of reflexology, I will bring this method to you.

You need no longer live in fear of so-called incurable diseases: nothing is incurable; diseases are the result of malfunctioning cells and imperfection of the body tissues due to unnatural elements of living. Just turn to nature and give her a chance to put your body chemistry back into normal performance by rebuilding perfect cells and new healthy tissues for your whole body.

How Rejuvenation Is Possible with Reflexology

Since time immemorial people have been looking for means of rejuvenation outside of themselves. They expected rejuvenation from witchcraft, the philosopher's stone, the fountain of youth, and so forth. The one place they forgot to search, where such possibilities have always been at hand, was within themselves.

RETURN TO YOUTH IS POSSIBLE

Who says we can't return to youth? Let me give you some facts of proof that it is possible to turn back the clock. I don't believe that man was meant to grow old and die so soon.

Prof. Hilton Hotema states, "Before the flood, men are said to have lived 500 and even 900 or more years. As a physiologist I can assert positively that there is no fact reached by science to contradict or render this as improbable. It is more difficult, on scientific grounds, to explain why man dies at all, than it is to believe in the duration of human life over a thousand years."

Ancient Masters Spoke of Rejuvenation

Some of the ancient masters often spoke of cases of rejuvenation, but their accounts have not been understood.

"His flesh shall be fresh as a child's; he shall return to the days of his youth. And thy youth shall be renewed like the eagle's. These things worketh God oftentimes in man when man knows how to live in harmony with the law." (Job 33; 25, 29: Psalms 103; 5)

The human body is a materialization of invisible gases of the air, consisting of electrolyzed and intelligized atoms. The person corresponds in color, number, and vibrations to the solar system at the moment of birth. A person (you) becomes embodied in a prison of matter and your mind is inseparable from cosmic elements.

Your Youth Can Be Renewed Like the Eagle's

Your mind can, and does, control your body, and as soon as you believe there is hope for your renewed health and you start using God-given natural ways to turn the clock back, then "shall your youth be renewed like the eagle's."

Dr. Alexis Carrel, who kept the cells of a chicken heart alive for 32 years, said, "An organ is not made of (external) material, like a house. . . . It is born from a cell, and the body originated from one brick that would begin manufacturing other bricks from itself."

How a Man Out-Hikes His Son

Frank tells of his dad using some kind of a stick to roll on his feet.

"I remember Dad sitting on the edge of his bed every night and rolling his feet on some kind of a stick. When I asked him what he did it for, he just said the doctor told him to.

"Some years later when I came home from the Navy, my dad and I went on a hunting trip. He could out-climb me on every hill we came to. Up he would go like a mountain goat, while I puffed along behind him, with rests in between. He kept saying 'Come on, what is the matter with you, Frank?" He was a lot younger than I was physically. And I noticed he still rolled his feet on the stick every night.

"When I was introduced to the methods of reflexology, I realized why my dad had been so energetic and healthy up into his late years."

Eighty-seven-Year-Old Grandma Falls Downstairs

I gave a friend, Lynetta, a book as a gift, and she said her 87-year-old grandmother borrowed it and never gave it back. "She thinks it is the most wonderful book she has ever read," Lynetta tells me:

"She uses it constantly on herself and everyone else including me, and it has helped all of us in many ways, yes, even the children. But let me tell you about Grandma falling down the stairs. She lives alone in her own house which has a basement where she does her washing. The other day Grandma came over and told me this story.

"'I fell down the steps the other day into the basement.' I was horrified, but I could tell Grandma was O.K. 'What happened?' I asked. 'Well, I opened the basement door and then turned to pick up some things I was going to take downstairs. I kind of got tangled up in some string on one of the boxes, and the next thing I knew, me and all those boxes and stuff were tumbling bumpety-bump down the steps.'

"'When I hit the bottom I just lay there a few minutes wondering if anything was broken. Then I started to wiggle my fingers and found out they were all right, then I wiggled my toes, then I started to rub my fingers and as soon as I could get myself untangled I also started massaging my feet. I didn't move from that floor for a good half hour until I had massaged every one of my reflexes good. Do you know I haven't even been sore from that fall? I wonder what I would have been like if I hadn't known about reflexology?'

"She credits everything to her reflex massage, and I will have to agree with her, it is the greatest thing that has happened to this family."

Always keep in mind that reflexology will absolutely relieve pain and, in most cases, remove the cause.

Nature has provided us with the necessities to sustain life and has generously given us this easy method of freeing ourselves from pain and ill health. Since we continually make use of all the other gifts of nature, we should gratefully accept her most precious gift, a healthy happy life through reflexology.

How Aged Father Maintains Health

A gentleman says, "Although my father is quite old in years, because of his boundless energy people find it almost impossible to believe his true age. Since reading about reflexology, I think I know the answer.

"Whenever he is sitting idly talking or watching television, he is constantly massaging his hands. He massages one hand completely with the thumb of the opposite hand pressed into the palm, while his fingers curl around and massage the back of the hand at the same time. He works over each hand in the same manner.

"I realize now that he is instinctively using one of nature's most marvelous gifts, the reflex massage method of achieving and maintaining good health. I believe this inconspicuous method of keeping a vital life force of energy flowing through his body is the secret of excellent health and long life."

How Schoolteacher Calms Nerves

Another gentleman tells us of watching his schoolteacher place the tips of his fingers together and press them hard against each other several times a day while he was walking back and forth before his class and while sitting behind his desk. He was using a natural instinct to calm nerves and keep the forceful life pulsations manifested in the glandular regions of his body. He will probably remain in perfect health all of his life.

Man, Ninety-six, Uses Reflexology Everyday to Help Himself and Others

Dear Mrs. Carter,

You may not know me, but I know a lot about you, and what you can do in your work of reflexology. I have been doing reflexology for twenty years. I have worked on people in eighteen states, many who have gone from one doctor to another, and could not get the help they needed. I have never had even one person come and tell me that it did not do them good. I am 96 years old now and still keep going. People tell me I have to live to be 120, because they need me here so much to help them stay well.

I did reflexology on a medical doctor, who told me that I helped him, when no one in his own line of work could. I worked on the reflexes of two people who had been to an acupuncture doctor, where they used needles to stick them, and this did not help. I helped them both feel better by using my fingers. I am in good health, I work on my own reflexes everyday to keep going.

Your friend,

Mr. E.S.C.

REJUVENATION BY MODERN PONCE DE LEON

An article in the Columbus, Ohio *Dispatch* calls a San Francisco physician, Baron Andrew Von Salza (who is now retired in Santa Barbara, California), a contemporary "Ponce de Leon."

Dr. Von Salza, a very good friend of mine, has helped me many times in my studies of natural methods to health. He is a specialist in rejuvenation, and studied the art of turning back the hands of time in Germany, Russia, and Italy. This modern Ponce de Leon was born in an ancient castle, built by his forefathers at the end of the nineteenth century in Thuringia, Germany. His parents emigrated to Russia where he studied at the University of St. Petersburg, then on to the University of Dorpat, Estonia, etc. The First World War interrupted his studies, but during the Second World War he worked in a biological research institute of experimental medicine that was created to study theories of rejuvenation. He worked with the highest specialists on the subject and with pupils of such authorities as Veronoff, Steinach, Alexis Carrel, and others.

After escaping into the American Zone, he developed a method of his own rejuvenation system, called J2 therapy. In his book *Return to Youth*, Dr. Von Salza tells us of many personalities, including T.V. and movie stars, who have returned to youth through his natural method of reversing the process of aging.

Woman in Mid Sixties Has Healthy Baby

As proof that the hands of time can be turned back, he gives this account of an Austrian woman of 62, about thirteen years post-menopausal. On the tenth month of treatment she started menstruation normally. On the thirteenth month of treatment she became pregnant and gave birth to a healthy child who is now 12 years old. The woman is now 76 years old, but looks to be in her forties. He gives many accounts of women and also men who actually returned to youth.

Seventy-two-Year-Old Man Regains Potency

He reports on Case #23, Male. High executive, 72 years of age, underweight—90 lbs at 5'5", no mental disturbances and perfect heart. Arteritis obliterans along lower limbs, acute arthritis, arteriosclerosis with pronounced muscular atrophy. Parchment-like facial skin. Unable to dress or walk, completely bedridden. Two years later: weight 110, no sign of arteritis obliterans, no sign of muscular atrophy, skin has healthy tan, very agile, got back his driver's license. Potency returned with unusual vigor, something not experienced for at least 20 years.

Famous Personage Dances After Treatment

Dr. Von Salza gives an account of his experience with reflexology. "Mrs. Carter's book on Reflexology is a welcome addition to the field in preventing ailments as well as relieving tensions and pains of a chronic nature.

"To test the worth of Reflexology I invited Mrs. Carter to demonstrate her method of reflex massage on a famous personage, a patient of mine here in Hollywood, and was quite impressed with the result.

"My patient was in her late sixties, she could not move from one chair to another on the day of the treatment. The immediate improvement was quite astonishing and the aforementioned lady went to a night club in the evening and danced.

"I have enough faith in this method of healing to ask Mrs. Carter to open an office with my own. I believe that this is a simple and harmless method to health, and from my experience with Mrs. Carter I believe all that she says about Reflexology to be true."

Rejuvenation Therapy Used by Renaissance Spa

Now we learn that a spa has been opened in the Bahamas, by Dr. Ivan Popov, using the same rejuvenation therapy to reverse the process of aging that Dr. Von Salza has been using with such great success. Many of our most noted stars and people of society have undergone rejuvenation therapy at the Renaissance Spa in Nassau with fantastic results. They are overjoyed when these revitalizing treatments actually "Return Them to Youth."

Reversing the Process of Age

I don't claim that reflexology alone will do what these modern Ponce de Leons are doing, but their experiences do give proof that reversing the process of age is possible. By stimulating the cells with the vital magnetic life force from reflexology, you, too, have a chance to Return to Youth.

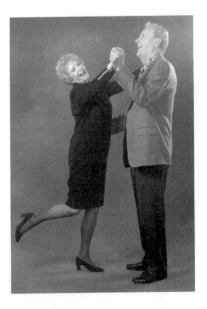

Photo 49: Reflexology is Nature's way to prevent premature aging and extend a healthy life!

REFLEXOLOGY IS FOR EVERYONE

Reflexology is a boon to all humanity. You can use this rediscovered art of healing, not only to alleviate pain and many ailments on yourself, but also on others. Do not be afraid to work any sore spots you may find on your hands or your feet; remember, *if it is sore, rub it out!* When there is pain any place in the body, follow the directions given in this book.

I am not a doctor, but through my lifetime of studying natural methods of healing, I give you the quickest and simplest method of helping yourself back to health through reflexology. All you have to do is press the reflex buttons in your hands, feet, or your body to start the healing forces of Mother Nature so that she may revive glandular activity.

Through the stimulation of these reflexes, you may be able to free yourself from pain and illness from this day on into your healthy happy future.

I give this book to you with compassion, knowing that it will reach out into the world and heal the anguished cry of deep despair and suffering. It is for all who will again turn back to nature for a way to live in perfect health the rest of your life.

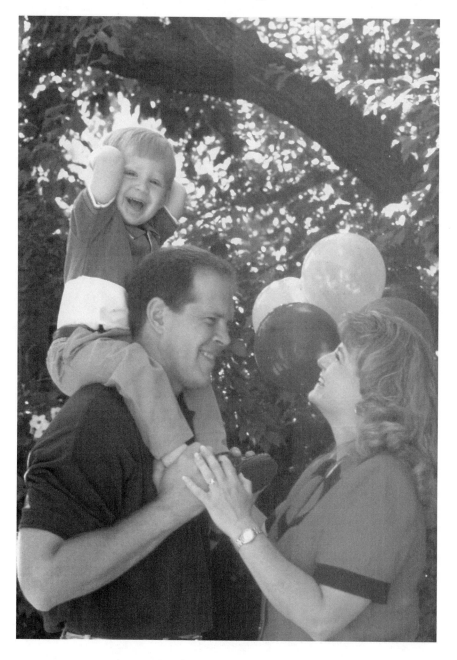

Photo 50: Now that you know reflexology is the key to perfect health, create a bright and happy future for your family and yourself.

Reflexology Photo Album

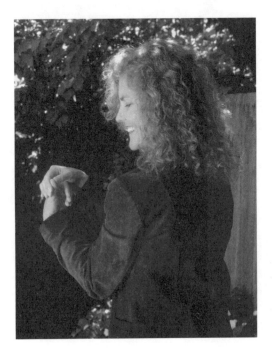

Photo 51: Stimulating the brain reflex for better memory. First work the upper pads of each thumb, then work the upper portions of all other fingers.

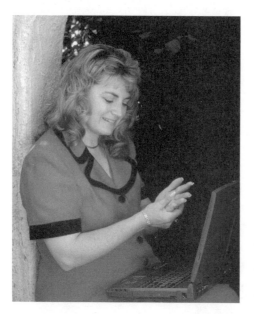

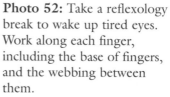

Photo 52: Take a reflexology break to wake up tired eyes. Work along each finger, including the base of fingers, and the webbing between them.

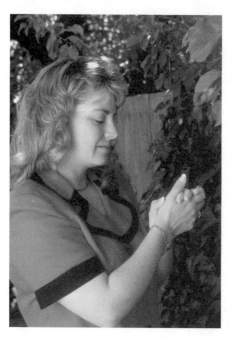

Photo 53: Position for working along edge of thumb to stop back pain. Also, work over zone two, around wrist, and up forearm. Repeat on other hand.

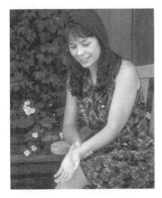

Photo 54: Position for working reflexes on the forearm to promote currents of healing energy to the lower lumbar area.

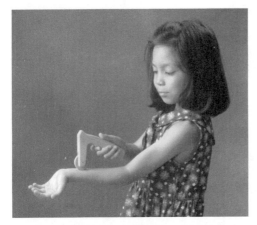

Photo 55: Shows the simplicity of using the reflex roller.

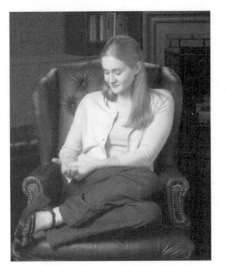

Photo 56: Working the thumb and fingers simultaneously on each side of the hand gives double benefits when stimulating the lung and rib reflex area.

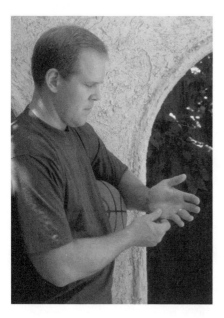

Photo 57: After sports, relax stressed shoulder and hip muscles, by working reflex areas along the outside of each hand.

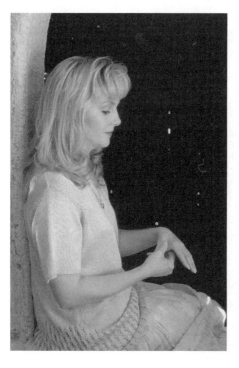

Photo 58: Working the Magical V on each hand is one of the most effective ways to restore health and revitalize the body.

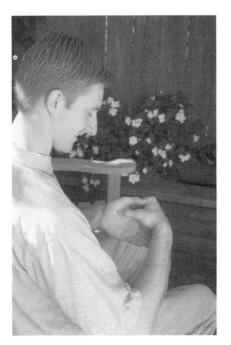

Photo 59: Working back-and-forth between the kidney, along the ureter, and the bladder reflex helps restore health to the urinary system.

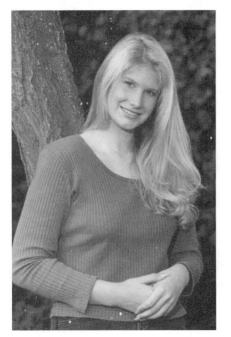

Photo 60: You can use reflexology anywhere. Even if you choose to use it discreetly, your body will benefit from the healing stimulation.

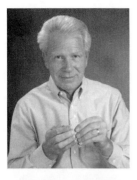

Photo 61: Release nervous tension by pressing the reflex comb on the ends of fingers. A steady pressure can reduce pain within the corresponding zone.

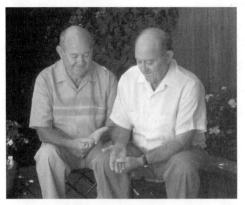

Photo 62: Twin brothers work the important reflex areas at the base of their fingers to help correct eyesight and improve hearing.

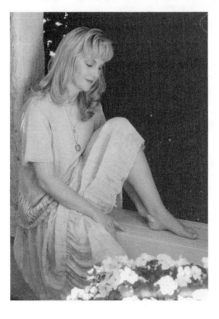

Photo 63: Using foot reflexology helps keep sex hormones in balance. With fingers and thumb, work just below the ankles on each foot.

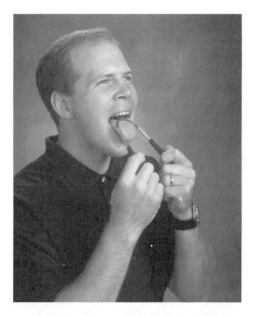

Photo 64: Scraping the tongue with a "Cleaning Wand" removes bacteria that cause bad breath and cavities, and it leaves the mouth fresh and clean.

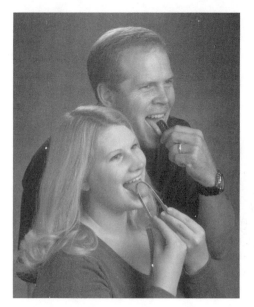

Photo 65: After cleaning, use as a pressure point stimulator on tiny reflex buttons in the tongue.

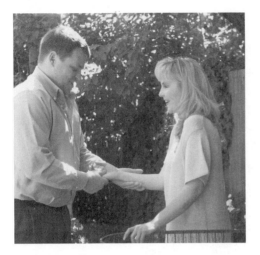

Photo 66: To renew your partner's energy level, vigorously apply rotating pressure on fingers, hands, and arms to activate and refresh circulation.

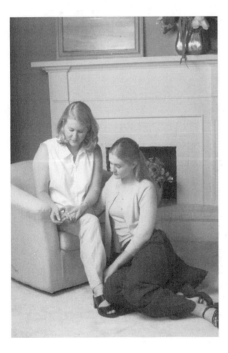

Photo 67: Sisters help reduce uptight emotions. Gently work the fingers, then with a firm grip, slide off the end of each finger to release mental anxiety.

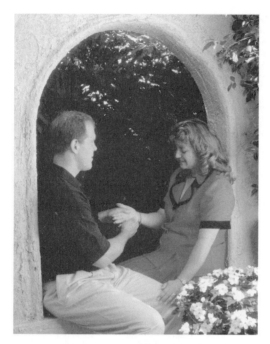

Photo 68: Reach out your hands and send healing energy into those you love.

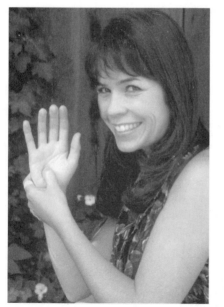

Photo 69: Position for working the colon. Using reflexology to stimulate the inner healing force is the first step to better health.

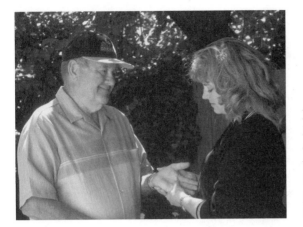

Photo 70: Daughter helps father with reflexology. It is nature's way to renew stimulation for natural and prompt relief from aches and pains.

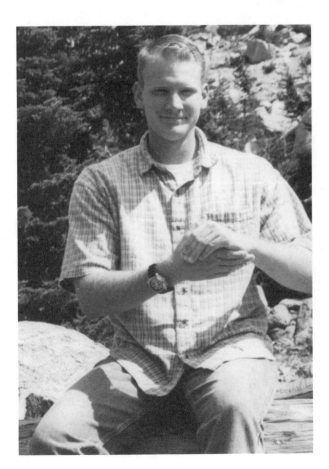

Photo 71: Reflexology is one of nature's natural healing forces.

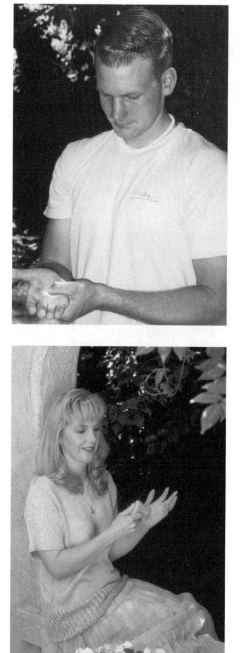

Photo 72: Using Reflexology is nature's "push button" secret for dynamic living, abundant energy, and vibrant health.

Photo 73: Reflexology stimulates healing circulation, which is important to renew cells and rejuvenate the whole body.

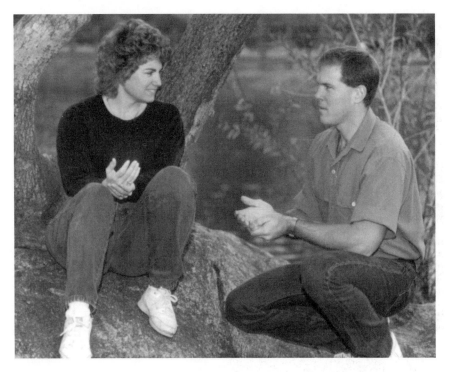

Photo 74: Reflexology is nature's way to better health. Try it today and see how it makes you feel!

Index

293

$13.00

DATE			